Current Diagnosis of Infant Tuberculosis Infection

Editor

Paulo Renato Zuquim Antas

Laboratório de Imunologia Clínica (LIC)
Instituto Oswaldo Cruz
Brazil

Co-Editors

Dilvani Oliveira Santos

Instituto de Biologia
Universidade Federal Fluminense (UFF)
Brazil

Roberta Olmo Pinheiro

Laboratório de Hanseníase
Instituto Oswaldo Cruz
Brazil

Theolis Barbosa

Laboratório Integrado de Microbiologia e Imunoregulação (LIMI)
Centro de Pesquisas Gonçalo Moniz (CPqGM)
Brazil

eBooks End User License Agreement

DEDICATION

This work is dedicated to tuberculosis patients and all health-care professionals directly connected to them.

CONTENTS

FOREWORD

In 2006 alone, worldwide 9.2 million people developed tuberculosis (TB) for the first time, of which 15-20% are children. The largest numbers of cases occurred in India, China and Indonesia, while the African continent, particularly sub-Saharan Africa, continued to feature the highest incidence rates (363/100,000 people). Approximately 1.7 million individuals died from TB; 0.2 million of which occurred in HIV-co-infected cases. TB continued to be the leading cause of death in HIV-infected individuals in Africa. TB predominantly affects young adults, and thereby hampers sustainable development in developing countries, perpetuating the poverty cycle. Aggravating the current situation is the rising frequency of multi-drug resistant TB (MDR-TB) strains, which are resistant to the front-line drugs isoniazid and rifampicin. Sadly, MDR-TB is an iatrogenic problem, preventable by adequate treatment and compliance. More recently, extensively drug resistant TB (XDR-TB) has emerged, with additional resistance to fluoroquinolone derivatives and at least one of the second-line injectable drugs (amikacin, kanamycin and/or capreomycin). XDR-TB has an extremely high case fatality rate in HIV-affected patients. Fears are that MDR- and XDR-TB may throw us back into the pre-antibiotic era, posing the threat of a virtually untreatable disease.

Thus, TB continues to pose formidable challenges to global health at the public health-, scientific- and political level. Our tools to combat TB are dangerously out of date, ineffective, or non-existent, such as easy non-invasive diagnostics for infant TB. Besides new tools (TB-drugs, vaccines, diagnostics), we also need new strategies to identify key *M. tuberculosis* / human host interactions, since it is here that we can most likely find *Mtb's* vulnerable spot. Equally important is that we build high quality clinical trial capacity and biobanks for TB biomarker identification. But most important is a global commitment at all levels to roll back TB before it outwits us again.

The current e-Book **Current Diagnosis of Infant Tuberculosis Infection** is a highly welcome addition to already existing scholarship since it uniquely underscores the relevance of all aspects of TB in the most vulnerable population of all: infants. This e-Book's scope ranges from basic immunology and microbiology all the way to clinical manifestations, diagnosis, treatment and management of TB as well as TB epidemiology. It cannot be overemphasized how important it is to bring TB back into the center of public attention, a place in which it should be in view of its horrifying consequences for affected individuals and populations.

Prof. Dr. Paul R. Klatser
Head of Department,
KIT Biomedical Research,
Royal Tropical Institute, Amsterdam,
The Netherlands.

Tom H. M. Ottenhoff, MD, PhD
Professor of Immunology;
Head Group Immunology and Immunogenetics of Bacterial Infectious Diseases,
Dept. of Infectious Diseases,
Leiden University Medical Center, Leiden,
The Nederlands.

PREFACE

One of the most extraordinary characteristics of *Mycobacterium tuberculosis* infection is its capacity to remain within the host's tissues for a long period of time. There is an enormous reservoir of persons latently infected with tuberculosis, estimated at about a third of the world's population. From this reservoir arise about 10 million new cases of active tuberculosis and more than two million deaths annually.

The natural history and clinical expression of infection due to *M. tuberculosis* differ substantially in children depending upon the age at infection and the host immune status. Children infected prior to age 4 are very unlikely to develop reactivation disease in adulthood, however, they have a very high rate of developing immediate clinical or radiographic manifestations, or both. In contrast, children infected in preadolescence or adolescence are more prone to develop more severe adult-type pulmonary tuberculosis soon after infection or in adulthood. Also, children with tuberculosis respond well to and tolerate the same basic treatment regimens as used for adults. Some prevention of childhood tuberculosis can be achieved by the use of the bacille Calmette-Guérin (BCG) vaccines, but the use of chemotherapy to treat recent tuberculosis infection, discovered *via* contact tracing, is of paramount importance even when BCG vaccines are used.

The purpose of this e-Book, **"Current Diagnosis of Infant Tuberculosis Infection"**, is to introduce the reader the main problems involved in the diagnosis of this disease, giving an overview of commercially available options while, unlike most reviews on the subject, also explore tools currently under development. Our goal is to provide a comprehensive overview and update for the reader, particularly for pediatricians. Furthermore we hope the text is of use to universities and research centers, as well as all interested hospital personnel. We believe that providing understandable and practice-oriented information on this subject, while keeping in mind frontier research developments, will help clinicians improve their diagnostic skills regarding tuberculosis infection in child. Each co-author provides the view from his/her field of expertise, benefiting from the experience of working with mycobacteriosis in the endemic country of Brazil. Brazil is one of the 22 countries listed with the highest burden of tuberculosis worldwide. We emphasize a knowledge-based product of the highest quality for the academic, professional, and student communities worldwide.

We would like to express our sincere appreciation to all of the authors who contributed chapters to this e-Book. We also would like to thank Bentham Science Publishers for their very kind support and efforts.

Paulo R.Z. Antas
Laboratório de Imunologia Clínica
Instituto Oswaldo Cruz, Fiocruz, Rio de Janeiro
Brazil.

EDITOR

Dilvani O. Santos
Laboratório de Biopatógenos e Ativação Celular, Instituto de Biologia, Universidade Federal Fluminense, Niterói, Brazil.

Roberta O. Pinheiro
Laboratório de Hanseníase, Instituto Oswaldo Cruz, Fiocruz, Rio de Janeiro, Brazil.

Theolis Barbosa
Laboratório Integrado de Microbiologia e Imunoregulação, Centro de Pesquisas Gonçalo Moniz, Fiocruz, Salvador, Brazil.

CO-EDITORS

List of Contributors

Almério de Souza Machado Jr. Assistant Professor, Escola Bahiana de Medicina e Saúde Pública, Salvador, Brazil

Dilvani Oliveira Santos Senior Professor, Universidade Federal Fluminense, Niterói, Brazil

Luíz Roberto Ribeiro Castello-Branco Senior Research, Instituto Oswaldo Cruz, Fiocruz, Rio de Janeiro, Brazil

Scientific Director, Fundação Ataulpho de Paiva, Rio de Janeiro, Brazil

Paulo Renato Zuquim Antas Research Assistant, Instituto Oswaldo Cruz, Fiocruz, Rio de Janeiro, Brazil

Former Assistant Professor of Parasitology, Fundação Oswaldo Aranha, UNIFOA, Volta Redonda, Brazil

Roberta Olmo Pinheiro Research Assistant, Instituto Oswaldo Cruz, Fiocruz, Rio de Janeiro, Brazil

Selma Sias Assistant Professor, Hospital Universitário Antônio Pedro, Universidade Federal Fluminense, Niterói, Brazil

Theolis Barbosa Research Technologist in Public Health, Centro de Pesquisas Gonçalo Moniz, Fiocruz, Salvador, Brazil

ACKNOWLEDGEMENTS

To **Tom Stuebner**

Center Director of Francis J. Curry National Tuberculosis Center, University of California, San Francisco, USA

To **Karen from Public Information Officer**

HPA - Communications 61 Colindale Avenue, London, UK

To **Jonna Petterson**

Public Relations Officer Nobelstiftelsen - The Nobel Foundation, Stockholm, Sweden

To **Gabriela Barbosa Zuquim Antas**

Cover design, pictures format and editing the images

To **Matthew Chapman**

Editing the text for grammar and fluency

To **CNPq Brazilian Grant Agency**

The editor is granted with a research fellowship (PQ-2)

2

CHAPTER 1

Introduction

Luiz R.R. Castello-Branco[1] and Paulo R.Z. Antas[2,*]

[1]*Instituto Oswaldo Cruz, Fiocruz, Rio de Janeiro, Brazil; Scientific Director, Fundação Ataulpho de Paiva, Rio de Janeiro, Brazil and* [2]*Laboratório de Imunologia Clínica, Fiocruz, Av. Brasil, # 4365; zip: 21045-900, Rio de Janeiro, Brazil*

Abstract: Of the 9.2 million new tuberculosis cases occurring each year, about 10% are in children less than 15-years old. Since childhood tuberculosis is usually non-infectious and non-fatal, management programs often do not prioritize diagnosis and treatment. Experts in childhood tuberculosis believe that children have been neglected in the worldwide effort to control this disease. Many reasons account for this apathy towards the disease in the young: The majority of children with tuberculosis are not infectious and consequently not considered to be as essential as adults with contagious tuberculosis, the lack of a microbiological diagnosis of tuberculosis in children, and the relative neglect of pediatricians and researchers in studying childhood tuberculosis. In fact, there is a rich scientific literature base regarding childhood tuberculosis supporting simple practices, which, if adequately put into place, would greatly improve the ability to diagnose and treat children with tuberculosis. This chapter will focus on historical aspects of this ancient disease plus parameters related to childhood tuberculosis, including the tubercle vaccine discovery and its first use in a French child. However, it does not focus on children and in particular on infants as we intend to introduce tuberculosis as a whole to students and professionals that are not familiar to the disease.

Keywords: Tuberculosis, Historical Facts, Robert Koch, Vaccine Discovery.

1.1. BACKGROUND

Although the exact number of annual cases of childhood tuberculosis is unknown, the World Health Organization (WHO) has estimated approximately 1 million new cases and 400,000 deaths per year in children due to tuberculosis [1, 2]. Most childhood tuberculosis cases are smear-negative, undiagnosed and untreated, thus given a lower priority in critical measures control; while many of these children could be saved if there were improvements in diagnosis and treatment available. The majority of children with tuberculosis are not infectious and consequently not considered to be as essential as adults with contagious tuberculosis. Lacking an established microbiological diagnosis of tuberculosis in children, while also the relative neglect of pediatricians and researchers in studying childhood tuberculosis, completes the sad picture regarding tuberculosis spreading in the pediatric population [3].

It is estimated that about a third of the world's population is currently latently infected with *Mycobacterium tuberculosis*. From this enormous reservoir arise about 10 million new cases with active tuberculosis, while more than two million deaths occur annually [4]. During the course of reactivation from latent infection to active pulmonary tuberculosis in humans, the first symptom usually perceived by a physician is an enlarging of an apical lung nodule on a chest X-ray image, which if removed and dissected, is generally found to involve Ghon focus with a central region of caseum and acid-fast bacilli staining. This specific characteristic is also often found in childhood tuberculosis cases. The most common way of acquiring tuberculosis infection, particularly during infancy, is by transmission *via* inhalation of infectious, aerosolized droplets nuclei or through the air. The bacilli enter the respiratory tract and into the lungs; then after a period of 4 to 8 weeks a primary pulmonary focus develops. The infection spreads to the adjacent lymph node and form the primary focus with involvement of adjacent gland, this clinical progression is

Address correspondence to Paulo R.Z. Antas: Laboratório de Imunologia Clínica, Fiocruz, Av. Brasil, # 4365; zip: 21045-900, Rio de Janeiro, Brazil; Tel: +55 21 3865-8152; E-mail: pzuquim@ioc.fiocruz.br

called the Primary Complex. In Western and developed countries primary tuberculosis occurs mostly in teenage populations, whereas in developing countries, infection may occur much earlier in life. In those adults who had developed primary complex in childhood, during periods of decreased immunity, the dormant mycobacteria can be re-activated with formation of cavities (or cavitation) in the lungs, which is called the Secondary, or Reactivation, Tuberculosis. Although the process of transition from latency to active disease is often not clinically apparent, it is well-known phenomena to clinicians with experience in tuberculosis, although they see it occasionally in earlier stages. Clinical observations and studies in humans provide insight into the components of true "containment". CD4+ T cell populations appear to be very important as HIV-infected persons with latent tuberculosis are at high risk of progressing to active disease. They frequently present with extrapulmonary or disseminated tuberculosis infection. Meanwhile, not only do CD4+ T cells limit dissemination, but they also promote lung inflammation. CD8+ T cell immune responses also appear to be important in healthy humans, particularly in maintaining latent infection. If not properly treated, or in non-vaccinated children, the disease then spreads to other organs of the body through the hematogenous route leading to tuberculosis of various organ such as brain (meningitis), other glands (lymphadenopathy) and even spreading to other areas of the lungs, like in miliary tuberculosis.

Established granulomas provide a niche where mycobacteria can remain viable, possibly dormant, in relative isolation from the host immune cells. Then they reactivate as the host ages or become weak. Recently, it has been shown that superinfecting *M. marinum* homes to established granulomas, suggesting that this niche ultimately favors the microbe [5].

1.2. THE DISCOVERY

Robert Koch (1843-1910), a German physician and scientist, made his famous presentation entitled *Über Tuberculose* on the evening of 24 March 1882, in Berlin. He began by reminding the skeptical audience, composed of prominent men in science from the Physiological Society, the terrifying statistics: "*If the importance of a disease for mankind is measured by the number of fatalities it causes, then tuberculosis must be considered much more important than those most feared infectious diseases, plague, cholera and the like. One in seven of all human beings dies from tuberculosis. If one only considers the productive middle-age groups, tuberculosis carries away one-third, and often more*". Koch's lecture, considered by many to be the most important in medical history, was so innovative, inspirational and thorough, that it set the stage for the scientific procedures of the 20th century. Using solid media made of potato and agar, Koch invented new methods of obtaining pure cultures of bacteria. He also developed new staining method, based on methylene blue, a dye developed by **Paul Ehrlich** (1854-1915) that counterstained with vesuvin, and demonstrated it for the audience: "*Under the microscope the structures of the animal tissues, such as the nucleus and its breakdown products are brown, while the tubercle bacteria are a beautiful blue*" [6].

Koch had brought his entire laboratory to the lecture room: microscopes, small flasks with cultures, glass slides with stained bacteria, dyes, reagents, glass jars with tissue samples, and slides of human and animal tissues preserved in alcohol. He wanted the audience to check his findings for themselves. Showing the presence of the bacillus, which he first named *tuberculosis bacillus*, was not enough indeed. He wanted his audience to note that bacteria were always present in tuberculosis infections and could be grown on solidified serum slants, first appearing to the naked eye in the second week. Furthermore, he showed that the disease that developed was the same, and the cultures of bacteria taken from the infected guinea pigs were identical to those inoculated tissue dissections gathered from different sources: Guinea pigs with tuberculous material obtained from the lungs of infected apes; from the brains and lungs of humans who had died from blood-borne tuberculosis; from the cheesy masses in lungs of chronically infected patients; and from the abdominal cavities of cattle infected with tuberculosis. Koch continued his speech, proving that whatever the dose and/or route he used, no matter what animal species he inoculated, the results were always the same: the animals subsequently developed the typical features of tuberculosis. He concluded saying that "*...the bacilli present in tuberculous lesions do not only accompany tuberculosis, but rather cause it. These bacilli are the true agents of tuberculosis*" [7]. When Koch ended his lecture there was complete silence. No questions, no congratulations, no applause. The audience was stunned. Slowly people got up and started looking into the microscopes to see the tubercle bacilli with their own eyes. On 20 April

1882, Koch presented an article entitled *Die Ätiologie der Tuberculose* in which he demonstrated that *Mycobacterium* was the single cause of tuberculosis in all of its forms. Since 24 March 1982, one hundred years after the seminal speech by Koch, World Tuberculosis Day has been celebrated.

The notorious Koch's postulates were then formulated in 1884, and finally polished and published by Koch in 1890. The postulates consist of four criteria designed to establish a causal relationship between a causative microbe and a disease:

- The organism must be found in all animals suffering from the disease, but not in healthy animals;
- The organism must be isolated from a diseased animal and grown in pure culture;
- The cultured organism should cause disease when introduced into a healthy animal;
- The organism must be re-isolated from the experimentally infected animal.

News of Koch's discovery spread rapidly. In 1890, at the 10th International Congress of Medicine held in Berlin, Koch announced a compound that inhibited the growth of tubercle bacilli in guinea pigs when given both pre- and post-exposure. It was called "tuberculin" and was prepared from glycerol extracts of liquid cultures of tubercle bacilli. Clinical trials using tuberculin as a therapeutic vaccine were soon initiated. The results were published in 1891 and revealed that only few persons were cured, at a rate not different from that of untreated patients. But, although results for treatment were disappointing, tuberculin was proven valuable for the diagnosis of tuberculosis [7].

One of Koch's papers [8], describing the preparation and partial purification of tuberculin served as the first description of the production of the partially purified protein derivative (PPD) of tuberculin, presently used in the Mantoux test, also known as the Tuberculin Skin Test (TST), Pirquet test, or PPD test.

Robert Koch was now a famous scientist and became known as "The Father of Bacteriology". He was presented with the Nobel Prize in Physiology or Medicine in 1905 "for his investigations and discoveries in relation to tuberculosis" (Fig. **1**).

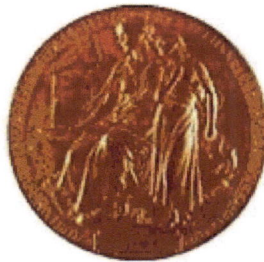

Fig. (1). The medal given to Nobel Laureates in Physiology or Medicine. Source: The Nobel Foundation.

1.3. AN ANCIENT DISEASE

Recent studies point out the genus *Mycobacterium* originating more than 150 million years ago [9]. DNA from *M. tuberculosis* in primitive tissues confirmed the incidence and spread of human tuberculosis in historic periods. However, the search for mycobacterial DNA in human archeological specimens has failed to find the presence of *M. bovis,* once considered a putative ancestor of *M. tuberculosis* [10]. Recent studies indicate that *M. africanum,* currently most commonly found in West African countries, might be considered a potential ancestor of the tubercle bacillus as well. Albeit Mycobacteria seem to be well preserved, the characteristic pathology induced in the host helps to strengthen the findings of residual microbial DNA contained in localized lesions. Those ancient materials proved that tuberculosis is an old disease with a wide geographical distribution. Thus, Mycobacterial DNA was promptly detected in the following sites below:

- Spine of a human from the Iron Age (400 to 230 BC) found in England [11];

- Andean mummies (140 to 1,200 AD) yield skin DNA samples [12];

- Calcified pleura (600 AD) found in the Negev desert, currently Israel [13].

Pulmonary tuberculosis is known since the time of **Hippocrates** by the Greek word *phthisis*, meaning consumption or "wasting away". This was the most used term and it is still used to name tuberculosis in different languages. Scrofula, a rare manifestation form of tuberculosis that affects the lymph nodes in the form of swellings, especially in the neck, most commonly found in children and usually spread by unpasteurized milk from infected cows, was well documented during the European Middle Age; it was believed that the touch of the sovereigns of England and France had the power to cure sufferers of the "King's Evil". Pott's disease or Gibbous deformity (Fig. **2**), a rare tuberculosis manifestation, revealed only among several antique Egyptian mummies, is a destructive form of tuberculosis that leads to serious spine deformities and subsequent member paralysis [14].

A   B

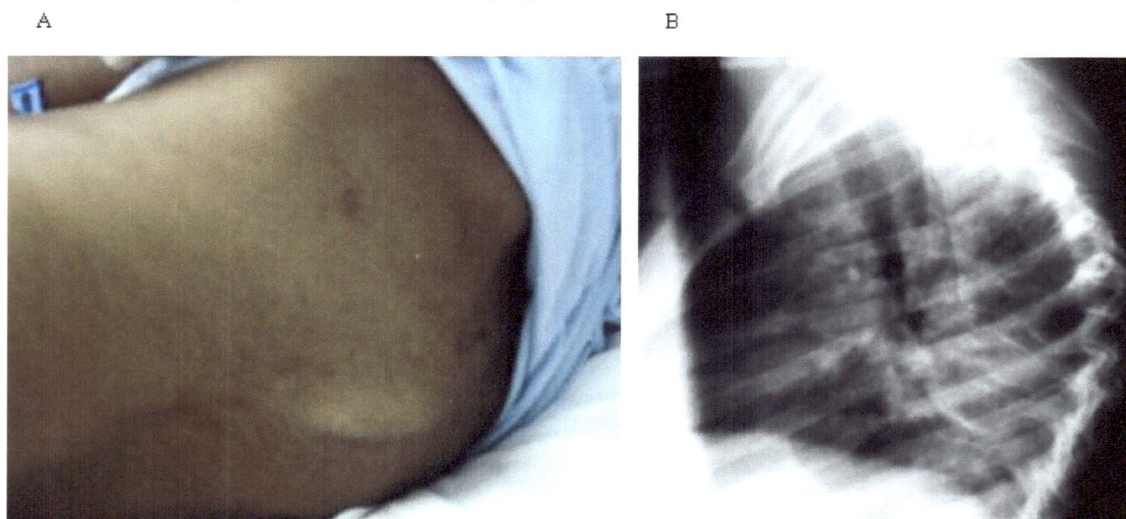

Fig. (2). (A) Kyphosis characteristic of bone tuberculosis in a 10-years old girl. (B) Chest X-ray image in lateral view of the same case as in A showing the vertebrae thoracic destruction. Source: Author.

The generic name "tuberculosis" has been used since 1840 to describe the disease caused by *M. tuberculosis*. The person responsible for naming the disease was Dr. Laennec. **René Théophile Hyacinthe Laennec** (1781-1826) was a French physician that is well-known for inventing the stethoscope in 1816 [15]. In March 1804, Laennec delivered a lecture in Paris, on the genesis of pulmonary *phthisis* describing that all the manifestations (infiltration, tubercles and cavities) were different aspects of tuberculosis in the lung. However, he did not realize that the condition was infectious. In 1839, **Johann Lukas Schönlein** (1793-1864) a German professor of medicine in the fields of therapeutics and pathology in Zurich, suggested that the word "tuberculosis" should be used as a name for the disease [16].

Regarding ancient treatment, heliotherapy was advocated as early as the 5th century AD by **Caelius Aurelianus**. Roman physicians recommended bathing in human urine, eating wolf livers, and drinking elephant blood.

Hygiene and dietary treatments were prescribed to patients as therapy for tuberculosis for centuries. Hippocrates recognized tuberculosis as a common and fatal systemic disease that localized mainly in the lungs. Treatment prescribed then consisted of resting, praying, drinking milk, dieting, exercising, and avoidance of exposure to inclement weather [17].

These treatments were based on spontaneous healing of patients under favorable conditions, as reflected by good food and, in the 19th century, resting in an adequate climate of the mountains as a key factor for treatment. This was possible through the establishment of sanatoriums (see below). **George Bodington** in 1840 produced a paper entitled "*An essay on the treatment and cure of pulmonary consumption, on principles natural, rational and successful*". This paper was the first to suggest the treatment of tuberculosis by a dietary, rest, and medical care. Bodington's idea failed for lack of support [18].

By 1650, tuberculosis was the leading cause of mortality. The high population density and poor sanitary conditions that characterized the enlarging cities of Europe and North America at the time of Industrial Revolution, provided the necessary environment, not met before in world history, for the spread of this airborne pathogen. The epidemic spread slowly overseas by exploration and colonization. In Europe, probably starting at the beginning of the 17th century and continued for the next 200 years, tuberculosis was known as the "Great White Plague". Of note, although tuberculosis existed in America before Columbus' arrival, it was striking rare among the natives [19].

In just 16 years, the face of tuberculosis has changed forever: From 1869, with **Jean Antoine Villemin** demonstrating that tuberculosis was contagious [9], through to 1882 famous **Robert Koch**'s speech, and to 1895, when **Wilhelm Roentgen** discovered the X-ray. All three were major achievements that were responsible, for the first-time-in-history, for a decline on the incidence of tuberculosis.

It should not be forgotten that **Pasteur** and other notable scientists provided important contributions to the theory of transmissibility of the disease.

The discovery of specific antibiotic chemotherapy, from the 1940s, changed the epidemiological profile of the disease; while in the 1950s and 1960s, treatment became primarily outpatient. In the following decades, most of the clinics for tuberculosis changed in hospitals for other areas of medicine or were even closed.

The antibiotic Isoniazid, also known as isonicotinylhydrazine, was later discovered to be effective against tuberculosis. It is manufactured from isonicotinic acid, which is produced from 4-methylpyridine. By mere coincidence, this was accomplished simultaneously in three pharmaceutical companies: one in Germany (Bayer) and two in the U.S.A. (Squibb and Hoffman La Roche). Concurrently, the drug company Lepetit Pharmaceuticals discovered that the mold *Amycolatopsis rifamycinica,* (formerly known as *Amycolatopsis mediterranei* and *Streptomyces mediterranei*), produced the new antibiotic Rifamycin B, later Rifampicin (*International Nonproprietary Name*) or Rifampin (*United States Adopted Names*). Other compounds with anti-tuberculosis activity were later discovered: pyrazinamide, ethambutol, cycloserine, and ethionamide.

Supervised treatment, including sometimes Direct Observation of Therapy (DOT), was proposed as a means of helping patients to take their drugs regularly and complete treatment, thus achieving cure and preventing the development of drug resistance. The Directly-Observed Treatment, Short-course (DOTS) strategy was promoted as the official policy of the WHO in 1991.

1.4. THE VACCINE

The Bacillus Calmette Guérin vaccine (BCG), was developed from a very virulent bacillus, *M. bovis*, isolated by **Nocard** from a heifer with mastitis in 1902 [20]. At that time, an important observation came from the fact that farmers milking the cows with tuberculosis did not develop full blown tuberculosis. After passaging the sample of *M. bovis* 231 times, *in vitro*, during 13 years at the Pasteur Institute of Lille, Drs. **Calmette and Guérin** noted alterations in the morphology of the colonies and a gradual loss of virulence. These cultures maintained the same physical properties and displayed continued immunogenicity in animal experiments, using chimpanzees, guinea pigs, mice, and cattle (Reviewed by [21]). On 21 June 1921, the first vaccination happened at the request of a French doctor, who wanted to protect a newborn child, whose mother died of tuberculosis after the childbirth, and who would have to live with the grandmother, who also had tuberculosis. Thus, Calmette administered BCG orally in three doses of 2 mg [22] and the child was reviewed for six months and did not show any sign of tuberculosis [23]. Calmette chose the oral route for his studies, as the gastrointestinal tract is the natural route for infection by *M. bovis*. Between 1921 and 1924, there were approximately 300 children vaccinated by the same researchers [24]. After the presentation of their results to the National Academy of Medicine in Paris, the Pasteur Institute of Lille was authorized to distribute samples of the bacillus to other laboratories all over the world. Between 1924 and 1926, at least 34 countries received the culture of BCG from the Pasteur Institute, while in 1927 another 26 countries received cultures of BCG [25].

From 1924 to 1926, it was observed at the Ulleval Hospital, in Norway, that the oral administration of BCG failed to produce allergic response and, in agreement with the incorrect hypothesis that the cutaneous tissue is an important source of antibodies, they decided to apply the vaccine parenterally *via* the subcutaneous route. It became evident that BCG was not deleterious and that parenteral administration could enable "allergic" reaction to the PPD [26]. Consequently, the intradermic route became popular, especially after 1927, when **Wallgreen** performed the intradermic vaccination; inoculating 0.1 mg of BCG in individuals of any age, negative to the TST. In 1930, Lubeck, Germany, a serious accident happened that caused profound changes in vaccination with BCG. Out of 250 children supposedly vaccinated with BCG, 73 died from tuberculosis in the first year, while another 135 developed signs and symptoms of disease [20]. Subsequent investigations revealed that a culture of *M. tuberculosis*, isolated from a sick child, was kept in the same incubator with the BCG and, during the vaccine preparation, the vaccine became contaminated. Calmette died in 1933, sad and discouraged after this incident in Germany. Still, in the 1930s, the institutional incorporation of new technologies to prevent, diagnose, and treat tuberculosis were adopted, with BCG, microscopy, mass radiography, and thoracic surgery all becoming prevalent (Reviewed by [21]). After the Second World War, the use of BCG increased in Europe and within the developing countries [22]. In 1966, as part of a WHO initiative the vaccine BCG started being lyophilized (Reviewed by [21]).

1.5. GREAT LANDMARKS

Hermann Brehmer (1826-1889)	A German physician who established the sanatorium cure providing the first widely practiced approach to anti-tuberculosis treatment. In 1854, he presented his medical dissertation *Tuberculosis is a Curable Disease*, based on systematic open-air treatment.
Edward Livingston Trudeau (1848-1915)	An American physician who established the most famous sanatorium in the U.S.A. He also suffered from tuberculosis in 1873 while in 1882, became aware of Koch's experiments with tuberculosis bacteria and of Brehmer's sanatorium.
Carlo Forlanini (1847-1918)	An Italian physician who discovered that the collapse of the affected lung tended to have a favorable impact on the outcome of the disease. He proposed to reduce the lung volume by artificial pneumothorax and surgery, methods that were applied worldwide after 1913.
Holger Mollgaard (1885-1973)	He introduced the compound sanocrysin in Copenhagen, 1925, which is a double thiosulphate of gold and sodium (Gold Therapy).
John Keats (1795-1821)	An English poet of the Romantic movement, who coughed a spot of bright red blood in 1820, and his life and his works became a metaphor that helped transform the physical disease *phthisis* into its spiritual offspring "consumption".
Alexandre Dumas (1824-1895)	A French author and dramatist who wrote the tale "The Lady of the Camellias" (1848) as the first romantic redemption.
Giuseppe Verdi (1813-1901)	An Italian Romantic composer of the famous opera "La Traviata" (1853) following the reflection of societal ills.
Giacomo Puccini (1858-1924)	An Italian composer of the opera "La bohème" (1896) that portrays tuberculosis in a new environment, affecting street artists struggling with poverty and disease.
Wilhelm Konrad von Röntgen (1845-1923)	A German physicist who earned the first Nobel Prize in Physics in 1901 when discovered the X-rays, a further significant advance in 1895 (see chapter 6).
Albert Calmette (1863-1933)	From 1908 until 1919 in France, they discovered the BCG vaccine against

and **Camille Guérin** (1872-1961)	tuberculosis (see above).
Selman A. Waksman (1888-1973) and **Albert Schatz** (1920-2005)	In 1943, two American biochemists and microbiologists discovered the streptomycin, a compound with antibiotic activity purified from *Streptomyces griseus* [27].
Jörgen Lehmann (1898-1989)	In 1943, a Danish-born Swedish physician and chemist observed that a drug called Para-aminosalicylic acid (PAS), very similar to salt of aspirin, had anti-tuberculous properties [28]. PAS was produced and first tested as an oral therapy at the end of 1944.
Gerhard Domagk (1895-1964)	A German pathologist and bacteriologist who received in 1939 the Nobel Prize in Physiology or Medicine when discovered in 1949 the first sulphonamide, latter called isoniazid [29].
John Crofton (1912-2009)	First employed the three-drug therapy (streptomycin, PAS, and isoniazid).

Adapted from [30]

REFERENCES

[1]   Kochi A. The global tuberculosis situation and the new control strategy of the World Health Organization. Tubercle 1991; 1-6.

[2]   World Health Organization. Global Tuberculosis Control. 2007. Report No. 2007.

[3]   Starke JR. Childhood tuberculosis: ending the neglect. Int J Tuberc Lung Dis 2002; 6: 373-4.

[4]   World Health Organization. Global Tuberculosis control: epidemiology, strategy, financing report. 2009. Report No. 2009.

[5]   Houben EN, Nguyen L, Pieters J. Interaction of pathogenic mycobacteria with the host immune system. Curr Opin Microbiol 2006; 9(1): 76-85.

[6]   Koch R. Classics in infectious diseases: The etiology of tuberculosis: Robert Koch. Berlin, Germany 1882. Rev Infect Dis 1982; 4: 1270-4.

[7]   Kaufmann SH, Schaible UE. Robert Koch's Nobel Prize for the discovery of the tubercle bacillus. Trends Microbiol 2005; 13: 469-75.

[8]   Koch R. Weitere Mittheilungen nber das Tuberkulin. Dt Med Wochenschr 1891; 17: 1189-92.

[9]   Daniel TM. The history of tuberculosis. Respir Med 2006; 100: 1862-70.

[10] Donoghue HD, Spigelman M, Greenblatt CL, Lev-Maor G, Bar-Gal GK, Matheson C, *et al.* Tuberculosis: from prehistory to Robert Koch, as revealed by ancient DNA. Lancet Infect Dis 2004; 4: 584-92.

[11] Taylor GM, Young DB, Mays SA. Genotypic analysis of the earliest known prehistoric case of tuberculosis in Britain. J Clin Microbiol 2005; 43: 2236-40.

[12] Konomi N, Lebwohl E, Mowbray K, Tattersall I, Zhang D. Detection of mycobacterial DNA in Andean mummies. J Clin Microbiol 2002; 40: 4738-40.

[13] Donoghue HD, Spigelman M, Zias J, Gernaey-Child AM, Minnikin DE. *Mycobacterium tuberculosis* complex DNA in calcified pleura from remains 1400 years old. Lett Appl Microbiol 1998; 27: 265-9.

[14] Ducati RG, Santos DS. The resumption of consumption: a review on tuberculosis. Mem Inst Oswaldo Cruz 2006; 101(7): 697-714.

[15] Laennec RTH. De l'Auscultation Médiate ou Trait du Diagnostic des Maladies des Poumon et du Coeur. 1st ed. Brosson & Chaudé. Paris 1819.

[16] The White Plague. Tuberculosis, Man, and Society. Rutgers University Press. New Jersey 1996.

[17] Rosenblatt MB. Pulmonary tuberculosis: Evolution of modern therapy. Bull NY Acad Med 1973; 49(3): 163-96.

[18] Keers RY. Two forgotten pioneers: James Carson and George Bodington. Thorax 1980; 35(7): 483-9.

[19] Bates JH, Stead WW. The history of tuberculosis as a global epidemic. Med Clin North Am 1993; 77: 1205-17.

[20] Sakula A. BCG: Who were Calmette and Guerin? Thorax 1983; 38(11): 806-12.

[21] Benevolo-de-Andrade TC, Monteiro-Maia R, Cosgrove C, Castello-Branco LR. BCG Moreau Rio de Janeiro: an oral vaccine against tuberculosis-review. Mem Inst Oswaldo Cruz 2005; 100(5): 459-65.

[22] Succi RCM. BCG. In: Farhat CK, editor. Fundamentos e Prática das Imunizações em Clínica Médica e Pediatria. Atheneu. Rio de Janeiro 1985. pp. 27-41.

[23]   Lagrange PH. Vaccination antituberculeuse par le BCG: historique d'une decouverte et de sus controverses. Medicin Sciences 1998; 14: 314-9.

[24]   Assis A. Estado actual da vaccinação antituberculose pelo BCG no Rio de Janeiro. 1932.

[25]   Oettinger T, Jorgensen M, Ladefofed A, Haslov K, Andersen P. Development of the *Mycobacterium bovis* BCG vaccine: review of the historical and biochemical evidence for a genealogical tree. Tuber Lung Dis 1999; 79(4): 243-50.

[26]   Heimbeck J. BCG vaccination of nurses. Tubercle 1948; 29(4): 84-8.

[27]   Schatz A, Bugie E, Waksman S. Streptomycin,a substance exhibiting antibiotic activity against Gram-positive and Gram-negative bacteria. Proc Soc Expt Biol and Med 1944; 55: 66-9.

[28]   Ryan F. The forgotten plague: how the battle against tuberculosis was won - and lost. 1st ed. New York 1992.

[29]   McDermott W. The story of INH. J Infect Dis 1969; 119: 678-83.

[30]   Tuberculosis 2007. Available from: http: //www tuberculosistextbook com/index htm 2007 (last access Feb. 2010).

CHAPTER 2

Natural History of Tuberculosis in the Human Host: Infection, Latency and Active Disease. Are these Treatable?

Dilvani O. Santos[1,*], Selma M.A. Sias[2] and Paulo R.Z. Antas[3]

[1]Laboratório de Biopatógenos e Ativação Celular, Departamento de Biologia Celular e Molecular, Instituto de Biologia, Universidade Federal Fluminense, Av. Barros-Terra s/n Valonguinho, zip: 24001-970, Niterói, Rio de Janeiro, Brazil, [2]Hospital Universitário Antônio Pedro, Universidade Federal Fluminense, Niterói, Brazil and [3]Laboratório de Imunologia Clínica, Fiocruz, Av. Brasil, # 4365; zip: 21045-900, Rio de Janeiro, Brazil

Abstract: Tuberculosis in children should be confronted as a seminal event in public health, as it refers to recent infections supported by direct contact with infected people, mostly adults. However, due to children seldom constituting an important source of infectiousness thanks to the small ratio of bacilli released or spread, they have a limited epidemiology impact at a global perspective. Furthermore only those cases with larynx commitment plus those ones with lung cavity are at risk for contagiousness. There are three pathways that lead to illness: the progression of the primary infection, the exogenous re-infection, and the endogenous reactivation, (which is usually the basis for the post-primary or secondary tuberculosis in adults). Indeed, the possibility that persons previously infected with *Mycobacterium tuberculosis* can be exogenously re-infected has been debated for decades. Frequently, children can present both the primary form and the typical post-primary tuberculosis form of the adult. Primary Tuberculosis predominates early in life, predominantly in highly endemic countries, since children are constantly exposed to the infectious sources. In contrast, within developed countries, the risk of infection is lower and individuals can expect to reach adolescence or adulthood without *M. tuberculosis* infection.

Keywords: Tuberculosis, Childhood, Infection, Latency, Active Disease.

2.1. BACKGROUND

Tuberculosis is an infectious bacterial disease caused by *Mycobacterium tuberculosis*, which most commonly affects the lungs. Tuberculosis, or "consumption" as it was labeled, was described for many centuries to be a major cause of illness, although the real cause was totally unknown (see chapter 1). In 1882, Robert Koch, first assessed the diagnosis while observing the bacilli in stained sputum directly isolated from patients [1]. During the 20th century, it became possible to primarily diagnose an infection with the tuberculin skin test (also known as Mantoux or Pirquet test) which utilizes crude extract from purified protein derivative (PPD). More specific diagnosis of the disease was possible by the introduction of chest radiography [2-4].

Tuberculosis usually spreads from person to person *via* droplets from the throat and lungs of people with active respiratory disease [5; 6]. In healthy people, infection with *M. tuberculosis* often causes no symptoms, since the immune system acts to "wall off" the bacteria. In such cases the infection stays dormant for extended periods of time, often for years. The symptoms of active pulmonary tuberculosis are coughing, sometimes with sputum and blood, chest pain, weakness, weight loss, fever and night sweats. Tuberculosis is treatable with a six-month course of antibiotics. Although tuberculosis is one of the major causes of death, infected people with effective immunity may remain healthy for years, suggesting long-term co-existence of host and pathogen [7].

---

*Address correspondence to Dilvani O. Santos:** Laboratório de Biopatógenos e Ativação Celular, Departamento de Biologia Celular e Molecular, Instituto de Biologia, Universidade Federal Fluminense, Av. Barros-Terra s/n Valonguinho, zip: 24001-970, Niterói, Rio de Janeiro, Brazil; Tel: +55 21 2629-2290 / +55 21 2629-2294; E-mail: santosdilvani@gmail.com

Paulo Renato Zuquim Antas, Dilvani Oliveira Santos, Roberta Olmo Pinheiro and Theolis Barbosa (Eds)

The natural history of tuberculosis is complex. Exposure of a healthy, uninfected, child to an adult source or index case of tuberculosis can result in an initial inflammatory reaction in the lung. This initial phase of primary infection with *M. tuberculosis* is also known as "Ghon focus". The Ghon focus may be visualized at the chest X-ray as airspace opacity and is commonly associated with a radiographically evident enlargement of the ipsilateral hilar or paratracheal lymph nodes (Fig. **1**). The combination of the Ghon focus and ipsilateral lymphadenopathy is called the primary complex or Ranke complex. In the setting of primary tuberculosis, parenchymal opacities may be airspace or interstitial in nature. Airspace consolidation is the most common radiographic pattern in primary disease. The most common interstitial pattern of primary disease is that of miliary (or disseminated) tuberculosis. Other primary manifestations of tuberculosis include tracheobronchial disease, hilar and mediastinal lymphadenopathy and pleural disease, *i.e.* empyema. In addition, adenopathy is particularly common in children with primary tuberculosis. However, pleural effusions are uncommon in children (10%), and may represent the only manifestation of primary tuberculosis, particularly in adolescents and young adults.

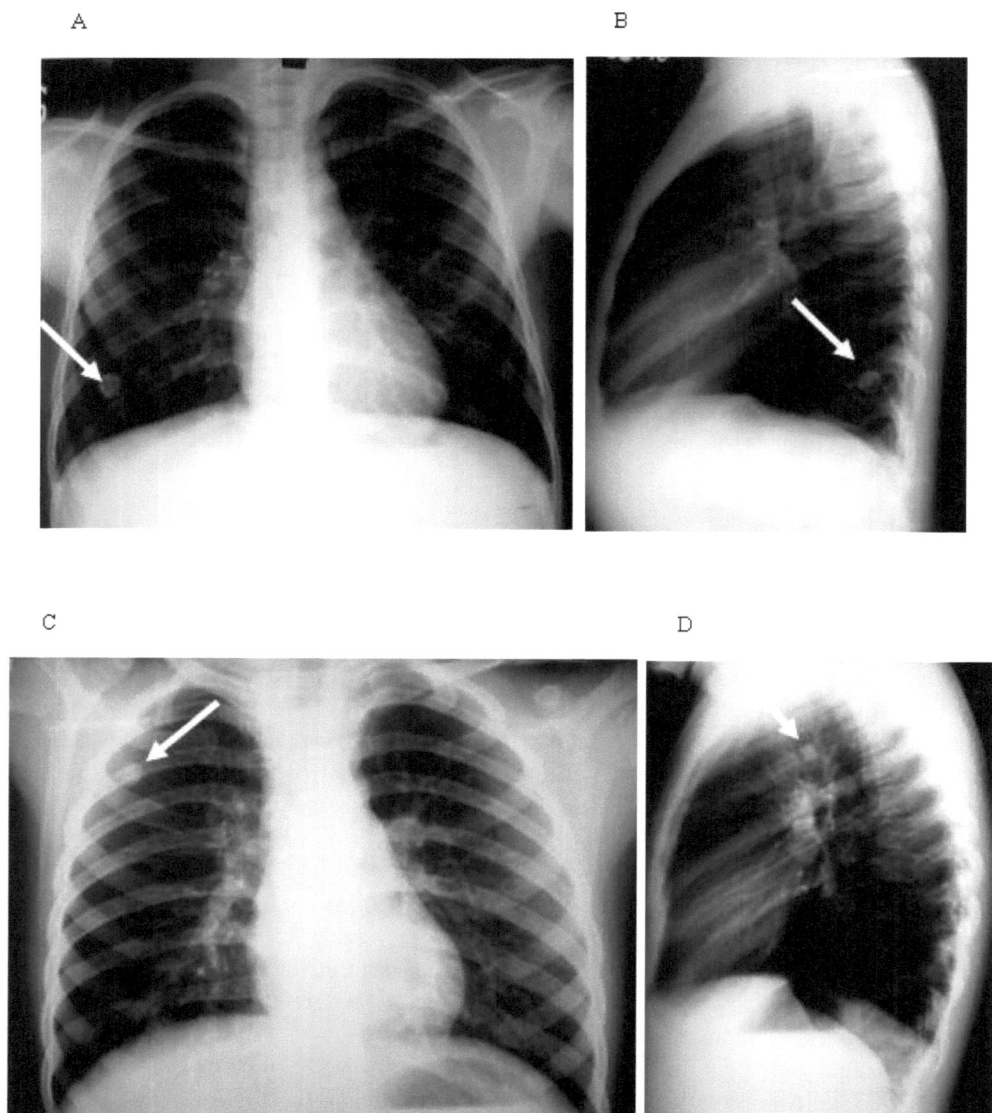

Fig. (1). (A) Chest X-ray showing the primary or Rank complex-calcified Ghon focus and ipsilateral hilar lymphadenopathy at the right lower lobe (arrow) of a 10-years old girl. (B) Lateral view of the same case showed in A. (C) Chest X-ray showing the primary or Rank complex at the right upper lobe (arrow) of an 8-years old boy. (D) Lateral view of the same case showed in C. Source: Author.

Also, a high magnification bronchovideoscope with subtitles (Available at: http://www.youtube.com/watch?v=xEAcSrv4_j4) shows characteristic tuberculosis patterns that can be found during assessment of child with suspected disease.

Children, usually less than 5 years-old, are more prone to develop active tuberculosis disease due to immature immune system, whereas elderly people, especially those with weak immune systems, become newly infected with *M. tuberculosis* and can rapidly develop active disease. In turn, this infection can develop either into primary tuberculosis disease or into a persistent, asymptomatic, infection that often remains clinically silent throughout life [2; 3; 7]. A latent infection may "reactivate" in about 10% of immunocompetent people and in roughly 8% of HIV-positive individuals each year, and cause symptomatic tuberculosis disease [7].

Children first become infected by inhaling *M. tuberculosis* (Fig. **2**). Thus, when tubercle bacilli reach the lung, the bacteria are deposited in the airways and alveoli in close proximity to the most ventilated areas of the organ; this is typically in the middle to lower regions (Fig. **2**). Although primary tuberculosis can affect any segment of the lung parenchyma, the lower lobes are characteristically involved more often in primary tuberculosis than in post-primary disease. However, this predilection varies with age. In children, it appears that the upper and lower lobes are involved with equal frequency, whereas in adults, there is a slight preference for lower lobe involvement.

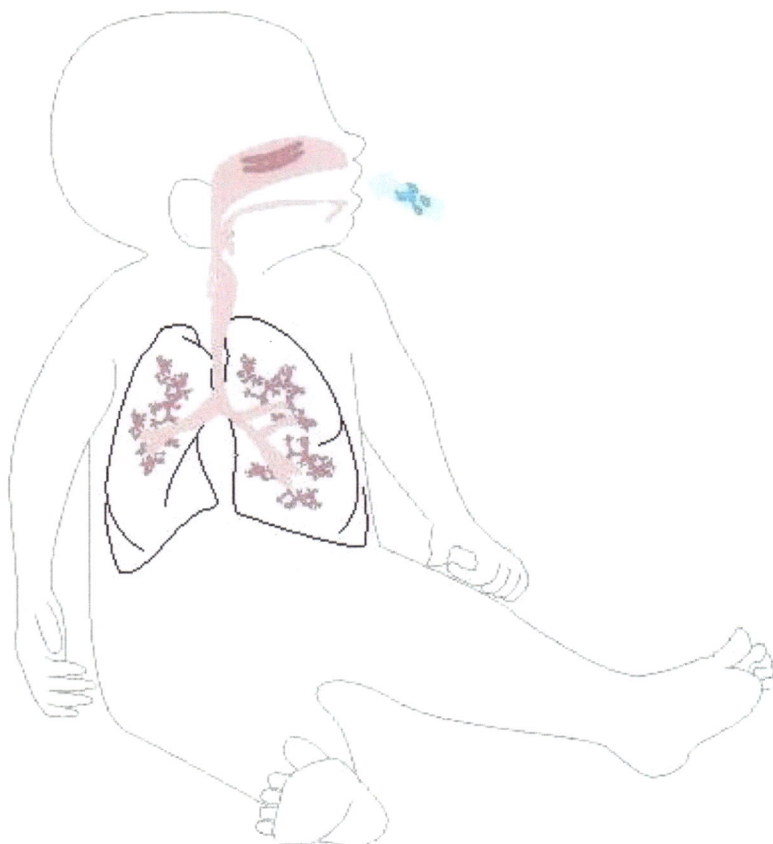

Fig. (2). Schematic view showing the primary way in which young people first become infected by inhaling the tubercle bacilli contained in small droplets from an index case of tuberculosis and thus reaching the lungs.

The crucial steps during the initial *M. tuberculosis* infection are summarized in the Fig. **3**. At the earliest phase, the alveolar macrophages in the alveoli of the lungs are the major host cells containing bacilli (Fig. **3a**), although pulmonary epithelial cells, covering a total of 70 m^2 surface area of the organ, can also be infected [8]. At this juncture, the bacilli begin to densely multiply, while other phagocytes such as polymorphonuclear neutrophils are also attracted (Fig. **3b**). If the individual fails to develop efficient cellular immune responses (see chapter 4), the infection of macrophages becomes the preferred course for the disease. Thus, *M. tuberculosis* can spread *via* lymphatics to the draining lymph nodes in the chest and result in enlargement of hilar and mediastinal lymph nodes.

In general, individuals develop prompt, innate and adaptive, immune responses to the bacilli. Furthermore, the development of cell-mediated immunity and delayed-type hypersensitivity, in most cases, result in host control of the infection (Fig. **3c**). The innate immune response starts during the first days of infection with vigorous release of molecules such as Reactive Oxygen Intermediates (ROI), to kill *M. tuberculosis* bacilli. Other molecules induced by cathelecidins produced by neutrophils, for instance the anti-microbial peptides LL-37, are also effective in killing the bacilli during this stage. Specific lymphocytes, such as natural killer and γ/δ T cells, also appear to play an important role during this stage of the infection. In most cases, the innate immune response is not sufficient to overcome the infection, leading to activation of other parts of the immune system.

The adaptive immune response starts with the activation of alveolar macrophages by the mycobacterial infection and, consequently, molecules called chemokines, such as CCL-2, CCL-3, CCL-5, and tumor necrosis factor (TNF) are copiously produced. The main purpose of these molecules is to attract T cells in a timely manner. Thus, specific CD4+ and CD8+ T cells initiate the adaptive immune response with the secretion of T helper (Th)-1 cytokines and mediators that help the macrophages to kill the bacilli. All these steps are orchestrated by cytokines released by the alveolar macrophages, such as interleukin-12 (IL-12) and IL-18. One of the major risks of tuberculosis is over-activation of the immune system and induction of pathology by severe destruction of lung tissue leading to the clinical symptoms [9, 10].

The future of such patient depends on the subsequent behavior of the caseous component of any active lesion in the lung. In most patients, the lesion becomes surrounded by fibrous tissue and the caseum calcifies, leading to a stable, encapsulated, tuberculoma (Fig. **3d**). In other patients, for unknown reasons, the caseous material undergoes liquefaction, the tubercle bacilli fully proliferate and express more antigens at the site of the lesion. This, in turn, causes a greater cellular immune response, and the lesion enlarges. Eventually, the necrotic zone may rupture into a neighboring bronchus (Fig. **3e**), the liquid caseum drains into the bronchus and will be replaced by air, resulting in a small tuberculosis cavity [11]. Nevertheless, cavitation is relatively uncommon in primary disease, particularly in young children. Current conjecture indicates that genetic factors are most likely related to the expression of the disease.

During the development of tuberculosis in children three stages should be considered: exposure, infectiousness and disease disposition.

Exposure implies direct contact with any tuberculosis patient, adult or adolescent, infected with active *M. tuberculosis*. At this stage, there is no clear evidence of disease and the tuberculin skin test is usually negative. Between two and twelve weeks after the contact with the bacilli the skin test becomes positive and thereby provides more accurate readings.

The infection is often characterized by a positive skin test reaction to tuberculin, however with normal chest X-rays. It can also present through calcified images at the lymph nodes or in the pulmonary parenchyma. The majority of children with primary tuberculosis infection have normal chest X-ray and they do not present clear evidence of clinical signs of disease (see chapter 6). Occasionally, unspecific symptoms are also observed, such as low fever, malaise and cough. Asymptomatic presentation can be found among school children, while less frequently with nursing babies of less than one year of age.

After primary infection, some individuals develop progressive primary disease. This form of tuberculosis may develop from any pulmonary or ganglionary focus, as well as from hematogenous dissemination (Fig. **3f**). It is currently speculated that factors such as the age and the nutritional status of the child usually determine the progression to infection.

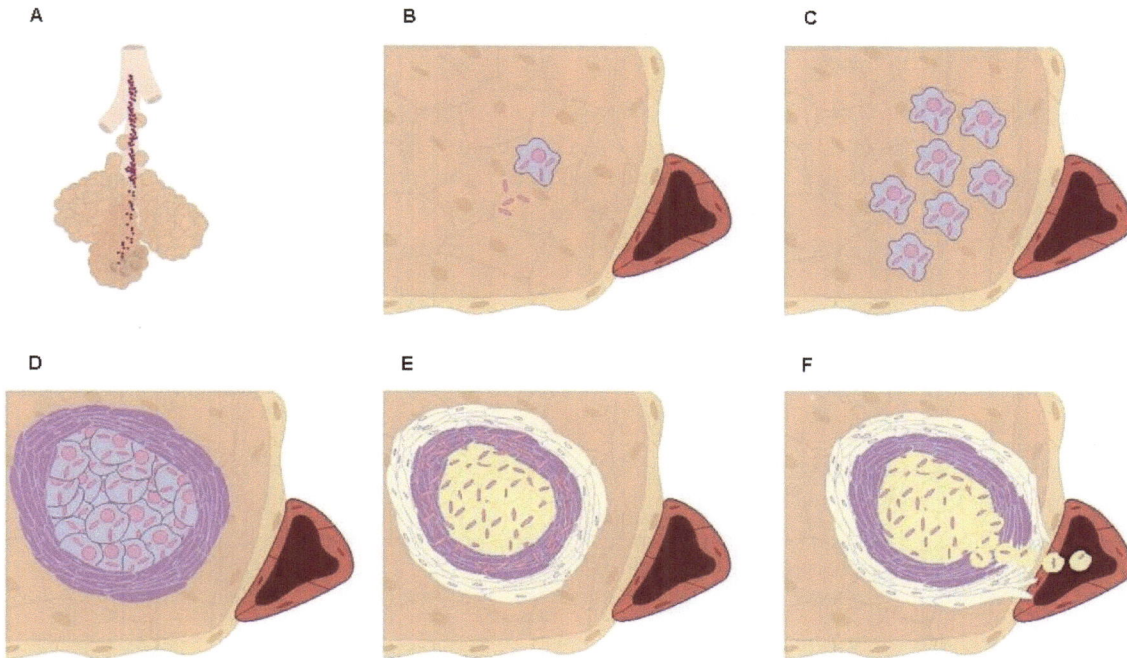

Fig. (3). Sequential scheme after the tubercle bacilli inhalation showing the moments (A) when the mycobacteria reach the alveoli of the lung, (B) the bacilli encounters the host phagocytes and (C) begin to densely multiply, thus (D) inducting lesion that becomes surrounded by fibrous tissue leading to an encapsulated tuberculoma, but (E) a central, necrotic zone that may be restricted to a calcified granuloma sometimes liquefies and (F) the liquid caseum drains into the circulation leading to hematogenous dissemination of the bacilli.

The healed lesions often contain viable bacilli that can progress to disease in the future. Such progression causes post-primary or reactivation tuberculosis. The post-primary tuberculosis arises in any individual that possess immunity induced either by natural infection or Bacille Calmette-Guérin (BCG) vaccination. Roughly 5% of recent-infected individuals may get sick latter either by recrudescence of a given latent pulmonary focus, endogenous reactivation, or by a new bacillary load, also known as exogenous re-infection.

The probability of an individual becoming infected depends on several criteria: the exposure to infective bacillary load, the virulence of the bacilli, the degree of hypersensitivity induced, and the natural or acquired immunity of the host. It is more easily translated by the Rich formula below:

$D = B * V * H * (In - Aq)^{-1}$; where:	**D = development of lesion** **B = bacillary load** **V = virulence of strain** **H = hypersensitivity** **In = innate immunity** **Aq = acquired immunity**

The Rich principle indicates that the development of tuberculosis damage is directly proportional to (i) the bacillary load, (ii) the virulence of inhaled strain and (iii) the development of hypersensitivity. However it is inversely proportional to both natural and acquired immunity. Risk of developing sickness is greatest directly after infection; however, it can persists later in life. It is estimated about one-half are at risk to develop the disease during the 2nd and 3rd years after tuberculosis infection.

It is important to point out that the distinction between primary and post-primary tuberculosis is of little clinical relevance. Active tuberculosis disease should be treated regardless of whether it is primary or post-primary in nature. Children who are suspected of having tuberculosis should be thoroughly evaluated for disease, including both clinical and epidemiological diagnoses.

Individuals are more prone to infection when they are young children (usually less than 5 years-old), aging people, immunosuppressed individuals or those tested negative for tuberculin skin test. Around 40% of the children with untreated preventive tuberculosis infection are more prone to develop active disease during the following one or two years. The age of the child and the time of infection are important to critically determine the nature and extent of the injury. The severity of the disease is greater if the infection occurs in the first year of life: While decreasing in severity into the 2nd and 3rd years thereafter.

Based on imaging techniques currently available, the following are the main aspects related to tuberculosis in children:

- The upper and lower lobes are affected equally in children.

- Radiographically, the primary complex consists of a parenchymal opacity and enlargement of ipsilateral thoracic lymph nodes.

- Involvement of the anterior segment of the upper lobes can occur in primary disease but is uncommon in reactivation disease in adults.

- The younger the child, the more commonly adenopathy is present and the more often it is seen without parenchymal disease.

- A lateral chest X-ray is often necessary to confirm the presence of hilar adenopathy in young children.

- There is a slight predilection for the right side, especially in the paratracheal and hilar areas.

- Enlarged lymph nodes may cause compression of airways leading to atelectasis.

Generally, tuberculosis is a disease of poverty, affecting mostly young adults in their most productive years. However, looking at the child population, tuberculosis history has to be considered differently.

In the past, tuberculosis in children was neglected because most pediatric cases have low transmission rates and therefore do not contribute significantly to transmission of tuberculosis in the community [12]. The new World Health Organization (WHO) "Stop TB Strategy", launched in 2006 [13], aims to ensure equitable access to health care to an international standard for all patients; regardless of age, gender, infectiousness or clinical condition (see chapter 3).

According to the WHO [14-16] the following are the main problems related to tuberculosis in children:

- *Diagnosis is difficult*: Effective procedures for tuberculosis diagnosis also used for adults, such as sputum smear microscopy and X-ray, are often not conclusive and need to be supported by additional tools;

- *Treatment is difficult*: Treatment regimens are different from those for adult cases, and their safety and effectiveness are not always fully documented. Not all anti-tuberculosis drugs are produced in pediatric formulations. Severe forms of tuberculosis such as tuberculous meningitis and miliary tuberculosis (also known as disseminated tuberculosis) are common in children. The clinical management of children with HIV infection or/and drug-resistant tuberculosis is more complicated than in adults;

- *Data are lacking*: In many countries, children with tuberculosis are seen by pediatricians outside the national tuberculosis agencies. National tuberculosis programmes consolidate and analyze their tuberculosis cases by age groups that are too broad to take proper account of children, and do not include the management of children with tuberculosis among their routine activities;

- *Prevention is neglected*: Vaccination of neonates with BCG and screening and management of household pediatric contacts are either poorly implemented or not properly targeted.

2.2. Management at a Glance

The incidence and prevalence of tuberculosis in children is increasing and becoming a particular problem in countries that are also affected by the HIV epidemic [12]. Tuberculosis in children has been seen as hard to diagnose but, at least in developed countries, relatively easy to treat. However, in children with HIV, severe disease is more frequent and this has led to a re-examination of treatment regimens [12].

In contrast, in adults the approach to first-line treatment of tuberculosis is well established. The success of the treatment depends on being able to provide a standardized short-course chemotherapy regimen with four drugs (isoniazid, rifampicin, ethambutol and pyrazinamide) reliably for 2 months, then 2, 3 or 4 drug combinations for up to a further 4 to 5 months, depending on the sensitivities of the infection and the circumstances of the patient, (especially the history of previous treatment). Adherence to the regime is critical to successful treatment. While use of fixed-dose combination products is recommended as standard care. Unfortunately, there are currently very few fixed-dose combination products available that are of good quality and formulated for treating children [14; 15]. In 2006, WHO revised its recommendations on the use of ethambutol in children, following an extensive review of efficacy and safety [15]. The outcome of that review was to amend the recommended daily dose of ethambutol for children of all ages to 20 mgkg^{-1}, with a range of 15-25 mgkg^{-1}. The process of carrying out that review and amending the recommendations highlighted two issues: Firstly, children metabolize tuberculosis medicines differently to adults, secondly, there was evidence available to inform dosage recommendations about "old" drugs. Neither of these findings are new, but the systematic consideration of them to inform WHO recommendations should be considered.

To ensure optimal treatment of tuberculosis in children, the dosage recommendations for the other first-line drugs required equal reassessment. In particular, pharmacokinetic studies of other first-line drugs needed to be gathered to determine whether current WHO dosage recommendations are likely to result in plasma concentrations that are sufficient for a therapeutic effect in children of all ages [12; 14; 15; 17-20].

Regardless of the above considerations, some questions still need to be answered:

- Can existing products be used safely and effectively in intermittent treatment regimens?

- What specific doses can be used in neonates?

- What should be the treatment regimens for tuberculous meningitis?

- What should be used in children co-infected with HIV and tuberculosis?

While more clinical trials may provide some answers, existing evidence should be used to aid refinement in the recommendations for these questions now. Furthermore, what is currently know, should help define projects going forward.

2.3. CONCLUDING REMARKS

Tuberculosis spreads when an index case who has active tuberculosis disease coughs in the air and the bacilli are then inhaled by another person. However infection usually requires repeated exposure to the bacilli. The entire course of infection to disease in a given individual is divided into five phases occurring at different times: Primary infection, primary illness, generalized dissemination, extra pulmonary tuberculosis and active disease. About 5-8% of infected people may develop primary or post-primary disease. Furthermore, while adults spread tuberculosis to children, it is highly unlikely that adults can contract tuberculosis from children as they are not able to cough with enough force to spread the bacilli in the air. Children are also at risk for developing more serious complications such as tuberculous meningitis, neurological disorders and permanent disabilities. It is likely that children who are infected with the tubercle bacilli will develop active disease at some point in their lives.

REFERENCES

[1]   Koch R. Classics in infectious diseases: The etiology of tuberculosis: Robert Koch. Berlin, Germany 1882. Rev Infect Dis 1982; 4(6): 1270-4.

[2]   Wallgren A. Primary pulmonary tuberculosis in childhood. Am J Dis Child 1935; 49: 1105-36.

[3]   Wallgren A. Pulmonary tuberculosis-relation of childhood infection to disease in adults. Lancet 1938; 1: 5973-6.

[4]   Wallgren A. The time-table of tuberculosis. Tubercle 1948; 29: 245-51.

[5]   Riley RL, Mills CC, Nyka W, *et al.* Aerial dissemination of pulmonary tuberculosis: a two-year study of contagion in a tuberculosis ward 1959. Am J Epidemiol 1995; 142: 3-14.

[6]   Stead WW. Management of health care workers after inadvertent exposure to tuberculosis: a guide for the use of preventive therapy. Ann Intern Med 1995; 122: 906-12.

[7]   Dye C, Scheele S, Dolin P, Pathania V, Raviglione MC. Consensus statement and Global burden of tuberculosis: estimated incidence, prevalence, and mortality by country: WHO Global Surveillance and Monitoring Project. JAMA 1999; 282: 677-86.

[8]   Wickremasinghe MI, Thomas LH, Friedland JS. Pulmonary epithelial cells are a source of IL-8 in the response to *Mycobacterium tuberculosis*: essential role of IL-1 from infected monocytes in a NF-kappa B-dependent network. J Immunol 1999; 163(7): 3936-47.

[9]   Narain R, Nair SS, Rao GR, Chandrasekhar P. Distribution of tuberculous infection and disease among households in a rural community. Bull World Health Organ 1966; 34(4): 639-54.

[10]   Stenger S. Immunological control of tuberculosis: role of tumor necrosis factor and more. Ann Rheuma Dis 2005; 64: 24-8.

[11]   Bloom BR, Murray CJ. Tuberculosis: commentary on a reemergent killer. Science 1992; 257: 1055-64.

[12]   Marais BJ, Gie RP, Schaaf HS, *et al.* The natural history of childhood intra-thoracic tuberculosis: a critical review of literature from the pre-chemotherapy era. Int J Tuberc Lung Dis 2004; 8: 392-402.

[13]   World Health Organization. Global Tuberculosis Control 2007. Report No. 2007.

[14]   World Health Organization. Global Tuberculosis control: epidemiology, strategy, financing report. 2009. Report No. 2009.

[15]   WHO European Region. www euro who int/childhealthenv 2010. Available from: www.euro.who.int/childhealthenv (last access Feb. 2010).

[16]   WHO European Region. www euro who int/tuberculosis/TBForum/20071002 2007 Available from: www.euro.who.int/tuberculosis/TBForum/20071002 (last access Feb. 2010).

[17]   Donald PR, Maher D, Maritz JS, Qazi S. Ethambutol dosage for the treatment of children: literature review and recommendations. Int J Tuberc Lung Dis 2006; 10: 1318-30.

[18]   Centers for Disease Control and Prevention. Emergence of *Mycobacterium tuberculosis* with extensive resistance to second line drugs, 2000-2004. MMWR; 2006. Report No. 55.

[19]   Friedland G. Tuberculosis, drug resistance, and HIV/AIDS: a triple threat. Curr Infect Dis Rep 2007; 9: 252-61.

[20]   World Health Organization. A research agenda for childhood tuberculosis. 2007. Report No. 2007.

CHAPTER 3

Epidemiology of Tuberculosis Infection in Children

Roberta O. Pinheiro[1],* and Paulo R.Z. Antas[2]

[1]*Laboratório de Hanseníase, Fiocruz, Av. Brasil, # 4365; zip: 21045-900, Rio de Janeiro, Brazil and* [2]*Laboratório de Imunologia Clínica, Fiocruz, Av. Brasil, # 4365; zip: 21045-900, Rio de Janeiro, Brazil*

Abstract: Tuberculosis remains one of the major diseases afflicting children throughout the world. The World Health Organization (WHO) recommends tuberculosis disease screening in children who live in the household of a smear-positive case, but lack effective measures for this management in high-burden countries to perform this routinely. WHO has recently called for more studies to define the global epidemiology of childhood tuberculosis, because the literature remains scant, dominated primarily by studies from industrialized countries and South Africa, but few epidemiologic studies of pediatric tuberculosis have been published from Asia. Children account for 10-15% of all new cases of tuberculosis worldwide. For a long time, childhood tuberculosis was neglected because of the paucibacillary characteristic of the disease in pediatric population. However, recent works have reinforced the role of childhood tuberculosis as an indicator of the effectiveness of control-programmes and also in the dissemination of the disease, since prevalent cases may persist for a long time. This chapter will focus on epidemiologic parameters related to childhood tuberculosis, including risk factors associated to disease development, the extrapulmonary tuberculosis epidemiology and the limitations in children tuberculosis diagnosis, which impairs the correct evaluation of the impact of tuberculosis in childhood community.

Keywords: Childhood Tuberculosis, Epidemiology, Risk Factors, Extrapulmonary Tuberculosis, Drug-Resistant Tuberculosis.

3.1. BACKGROUND

Tuberculosis has increased rapidly over the past three decades worldwide, especially in HIV endemic countries and in Africa and Asia. Increased international travel behavior and immigration have led to a rise in childhood tuberculosis rates even in traditionally low burden, industrialized settings, and threaten to promote the emergence and spread of multidrug-resistant strains. Whereas intense efforts to control tuberculosis in adults, childhood tuberculosis has been relatively neglected. However, children are particularly vulnerable to severe disease and death following infection and may be a reservoir for future transmission, following disease reactivation, in adulthood.

The latest estimates of the global burden of tuberculosis show that there were 9.27 million new cases in 2007 (including 1.37 million cases among HIV-positive people), of which 80% were in just 22 countries. There were a total of 1.32 million deaths from tuberculosis in HIV-negative people, with an additional 0.46 million tuberculosis deaths in HIV-positive people. This, in turn, equates to about 4,800 deaths a day, and 13.7 million prevalent cases (of which 687,000 were HIV-positive cases). The great majority of tuberculosis deaths are in the developing world, with more than half occurring in Asia [1; 2]. Per capita, the global tuberculosis incidence rate is falling, but the rate of decline is very slow (less than 1%). Tuberculosis is a worldwide pandemic. Among the 15 countries with the highest estimated tuberculosis incidence rates, 13 are in Africa, while half of all new cases are in six Asian countries (Bangladesh, China, India, Indonesia, Pakistan and the Philippines) [1; 2]. The classic age distribution of tuberculosis has changed, moving from a peak of over 50 to a median age of under 30 years old [3]. In general, children make up only a small proportion of cases, but in some high-incidence countries up to 15% of all tuberculosis cases occur in the pediatric population [4]. The HIV epidemic has caused a marked increase in the incidence of sputum smear-positive tuberculosis and a decrease in the peak age prevalence. The change in epidemiology has already resulted in an increase in the proportion of women of child bearing age contracting tuberculosis (40% increase in the U.S.A. between 1985 and 1992) and is likely to impact on the incidence of perinatal tuberculosis [5].

*Address correspondence to Roberta O. Pinheiro:** Leprosy Laboratory, Fiocruz, Av. Brasil, # 4365; zip: 21045-900, Rio de Janeiro, Brazil; Fax: +55 21 2270-9997, E-mail: rolmo@ioc.fiocruz.br

Perinatal tuberculosis is the term used to describe tuberculosis acquired in utero, intrapartum or during the early newborn period and is extremely rare if the mother is effectively treated in pregnancy. Although unusual (about 300 cases of perinatal tuberculosis have been described in the literature, in case reports, case series and reviews). Perinatal tuberculosis is believed to be increasing alongside a rise in tuberculosis incidence.

The data of global prevalence of tuberculosis in children are sparse and recent guidelines from World Health Organization (WHO) established that national tuberculosis programmes should report tuberculosis in children [6]. The 2006 WHO Global Report estimates that there are approximately one million cases of tuberculosis disease and 400,000 deaths each year in children above 15 years-old [6]. However, these data are underestimated since most data are derived from estimates of incidence, and most children have culture-negative tuberculosis. Fewer than 15% of children with culture-proven tuberculosis will be sputum smear positive, with the result that only a small percentage of children with tuberculosis will be represented in WHO data. Prevalent cases may remain undetected for prolonged periods, during which time they actively contribute to tuberculosis transmission within the community [7]. In addition, the occurrence of extrapulmonary tuberculosis (20-30% of caseload in some settings) is not described in most published figures of the burden of childhood tuberculosis [8].

3.2. RISK FACTORS ASSOCIATED TO SYMPTOMATIC TUBERCULOSIS IN CHILDREN

Epidemiologically, the risk factors and disease vary between industrialized and low- and middle-income countries. In industrialized countries, childhood tuberculosis constitutes about 2-7% of all cases, with many cases detected through contact tracing, and low death and high treatment completion rates being seen. This is in contrast to low- and middle-income countries, where childhood tuberculosis constitutes about 15-40% of all cases, existing in close association with poverty, crowding and malnutrition; few cases are identified by contact tracing, and there are higher tuberculosis deaths, but low treatment success rates [9]. In addition, other factors, such as family size, population density and the median age of tuberculosis patients in a given setting will determine the number of secondary infections per infectious case [10].

The annual risk of tuberculosis infection (ARI) is calculated based on tuberculin surveys of children 0-9 years-old, although this has limitations resulting from the poor specificity of the tuberculin skin test (TST), particularly where Bacille Calmette-Guérin (BCG) vaccine is given at birth and non-tuberculous mycobacteria are endemic. The ARI helps to determine the extent of transmission in the community as well as the efficacy of disease control activities such as case-finding and success of treatment.

Children who are in contact with individuals with infectious tuberculosis are at high risk of developing tuberculosis [11]. A study among household contacts showed an increased proportion of infected child contacts around a sputum-positive case compared with contacts of sputum-negative patients or households not including a person with tuberculosis [12]. Recent studies in sub-Saharan Africa have highlighted the importance of proximity of contact with female cases (mothers, aunts, grandmothers) with tuberculosis and risk of infection among children [13]. Despite the former vaccination with BCG, it has been suggested that a positive TST in a child who has close contact with an adult with infectious tuberculosis most likely represents real infection with *M. tuberculosis*, and treatment of this latent infection should be considered, especially if the child is younger than 5 years-old [14]. Children develop disease sooner after infection than adults, and thus the occurrence of disease in children provides an early assessment of transmission of tuberculosis within communities. Tuberculosis in children remains a sentinel indicator of the effectiveness of tuberculosis-control programmes [15-17]. According to Marais and colleagues (2007) [18] the most important determinants of a child's risk of developing tuberculosis after primary infection are age, with the highest risk occurring in children with an immature immune system (children < 3 years-old) (Table 1), and the immune status of the child. Most children who develop symptomatic tuberculosis do so within 6-12 months of infection, and active disease is most common under 5 years-old [19].

Table 1. Age-Specific Risk to Progress to Disease Following Infection in Immune-Competent Children.

Age at primary infection	Site of infection	Risk to progress to disease
< 1 year	**Pulmonary disease**	30-40%
	Disseminated disease or Meningitis	10-20%
1-2 years	**Pulmonary disease**	10-20%
	Disseminated disease or Meningitis	2-5%
2-5 years	**Pulmonary disease**	5%
	Disseminated disease or Meningitis	0.5%
5-10 years	**Pulmonary disease**	2%
	Disseminated disease or Meningitis	<0.5%
>10 years	**Pulmonary disease**	10-20%
	Disseminated disease or Meningitis	<0.5%

Adapted from [18].

Children account for 10-15% of all new cases of tuberculosis worldwide with marked regional and demographic variability [9]. Even in countries with low tuberculosis prevalence, rates of disease differ between urban and non-urban settings. Refugees and economic migrants are high-risk populations for tuberculosis, particularly if they originate from countries with a high incidence of disease [20; 21]. Childhood tuberculosis case rates in the United States are higher among ethnic and racial minority groups and the foreign born than in the American born Caucasian community. Estimates indicate, that in 2004, childhood tuberculosis accounted for 10% of all new cases in Africa and 2% in the established market economies [22].

Childhood tuberculosis is usually paucibacillary, although children are more likely to develop disease after infection and are significantly more likely to develop extrapulmonary and severe disseminated disease than adults [23]. In immune competent children, the risk of disseminated disease, including tuberculous meningitis, is age dependent, ranging from 20% during infancy to <0.5% in children 5 years of age, or older [15]. Several studies in countries with high HIV infection rates, however, have shown an increasing proportion of children with tuberculosis who are seropositive and thus leading to higher mortality rates [24, 25]. HIV-infected children are more likely to develop disseminated forms of tuberculosis and may develop immune reconstitution syndromes and complex drug interactions. The high prevalence of tuberculosis and HIV infection among adults in their reproductive years implies that children are at risk for both tuberculosis and HIV infection, and those seropositive children are more likely to be exposed to tuberculosis than are HIV-uninfected children [18].

A necropsy study in Zambia found evidence of tuberculosis in 32 (18%) of 180 HIV-positive and 22 (26%) of 84 HIV-negative children who died of pneumonia [26]. Among HIV-infected children aged over 12 months in a study from Zambia, tuberculosis accounted for 32% of deaths [26]. Also, tuberculosis was found to be the third most common cause of death in HIV-infected children with a clinical diagnosis of acute severe pneumonia [27]. Children who develop active tuberculosis often do so within several months after initial infection and, since infection in children is usually recent, prompt diagnosis and treatment of asymptomatic infection are essential. The risk of progression to active tuberculosis is highest in children younger than 3 years-old and approaches 40% in infants, with a second peak occurring in late adolescence [28; 29]. Surveillance data from the pre-chemotherapy era suggest that most children developed radiological abnormalities following infection, including 60-80% of children under 2 years-old; however, less than 10% of these were notified, suggesting that disease was controlled by the host immune response in most cases [15].

A study conducted in Western Cape Province, South Africa, described that children and adolescents with diabetes would appear to have 6.8-fold higher prevalence of tuberculosis disease [30]. That study showed a prevalence of tuberculosis disease of 4,242 $100,000^{-1}$ in children aged 0-14 years-old. Although this prevalence was higher when compared to non-diabetic pediatric population living in Western Cape (620 $100,000^{-1}$), the prevalence of tuberculosis infection in diabetes children and adolescents did not differ from that found in historical controls (non-diabetic Western Cape pediatric population, 30%) [30].

Additional factors that are associated with an excess risk of tuberculosis infection in children include malignancy, peritoneal dialysis and passive smoking [31]. A summary of risk factors related to tuberculosis disease in children is depicted below:

Poverty / Economic migrants

Malnutrition

Family size

Sputum-positive household contact

Immune status of the child

HIV and other immunosuppressive disorders

Peritoneal dialysis

Passive smoking

3.3. LIMITATIONS IN CHILDREN TUBERCULOSIS DIAGNOSIS AND THE IMPACT ON EPIDEMIOLOGIC EVALUATION

Smear-positive disease in children is less common than in adults, and thus a definitive diagnosis is more difficult to achieve. Presumptive diagnosis are frequently made and treatment is initialized based on exposure to an infectious adult case, a positive TST, and either a typical clinical syndrome or an abnormal chest X-ray [32]. Diagnostic uncertainty has been compounded by the HIV epidemic in which chronic lung disease, anergy, coexisting malnutrition and nonspecific clinical and radiological signs make definitive diagnosis even more challenging [33]. Until recently, only smear-positive cases were reported for children under the WHO directly observed treatment, short course (DOTS) strategy, yet smears are seldom done in many high-burden settings and most disease in children use to be smear-negative. The inherent difficulties in establishing a diagnosis of tuberculosis in children and the fact that children are not considered a public health risk are obstacles to the accurate estimate of the burden of disease. Because of these issues, the International Union Against Tuberculosis and Lung Diseases has stated that reliable information on the incidence of tuberculosis in childhood can only be obtained in developed countries, which have better diagnostic and reporting systems [34].

Case notifications of childhood tuberculosis depend on the intensity of the epidemic, the age structure of the population, the available diagnostic tools and the extent of routine contact tracing. However, epidemiological data on tuberculosis in children in high-burden countries are scarce [35]. Disease burden estimates, derived from assessments of the proportion of cases that are smear positive by age, suggest that children accounted for nearly 900,000 (11%) cases globally in 2000. Most of those cases occurred in 22 high-burden countries, where a combination of high transmission rates and a large proportion of the population under the age of 15 years-old mean that children account for up to 25-40% of cases, with incidence rates for pediatric tuberculosis ranging from 60 to 600 per 100,000 children per year (reviewed by (17]. One can estimate that, in a general population of 10 million (with 45% of children aged 0-14 years-old) exposed to a risk of infection of 1%, 45,000 annual infections occur in children, with 4,500 (10%) developing active tuberculosis disease; this ultimately leads to an incidence of 45 active cases per 100,000 population [36].

In the U.S.A. in 2001, childhood tuberculosis accounted for 5.8% of all cases of this disease, with regional differences due to an increase in population as well as to a large number of immigrants from high-burden countries [37]. In Peru, the case rates of childhood tuberculosis have declined from 12.5% in 1994 to 10.5% of all cases in 2000 [38].

In Europe, the rates of tuberculosis for both adults and children have been increasing steadily in the last decade. Furthermore, the overall case notifications reveal that there are some disparities in the rates of tuberculosis between countries in Western Europe and those in Eastern Europe. Rates of tuberculosis are very high in Eastern Europe, although age-specific rates are not available for all countries. Between 1999 and 2002, almost two thirds of tuberculosis notifications in Europe for children aged 0-14 years-old occurred in Eastern European region with 12-13,000 cases per year reported. In 2004, Kazakhstan reported more tuberculosis cases than the entire European Union for children aged 5-14 years-old [39].

In Western Europe, resources to fund tuberculosis-control programmes are available. Childhood tuberculosis cases in Western Europe were associated with the fact that children were born outside of the country, or had at least one parent who has born abroad. This is in stark contrast to Eastern Europe, where nearly all childhood tuberculosis occurs in children born locally [40]. In London, cases in children less than 16 years of age have risen almost every year since 1988. However, this was related to the increase of African children, with 95% of tuberculosis cases in this group residing in London [41]. Also, in Stockholm the overall rates of tuberculosis in children increased from <1 per 100,000 in 1976 to 5.8 per 100,000 between 1991 and 1995. This increase in case notifications was mostly due to children born outside the country (50% of children with tuberculosis were from Africa). There were no cases of tuberculosis in children whose parents were both Swedish-born from 1991 to 1995 [42]. In addition, a study in Copenhagen revealed that 70% of children with tuberculosis had immigrant parents [43].

In India, of the 245,051 new smear-positive pulmonary tuberculosis cases started on treatment under the Revised National Tuberculosis Control Program in 2002, 4,159 (1.7%) were aged 0-14 years-old, whereas a survey of the agenda implementing districts during the same year revealed that pediatric cases made up 3% of the total load of new cases registered [44].

3.4. EPIDEMIOLOGY OF EXTRAPULMONARY TUBERCULOSIS IN CHILDREN

Children less than 5 years-old are at higher risk of developing disseminated forms of tuberculosis, including miliary disease and meningitis, which are frequently associated with greater morbidity and mortality. A comprehensive review of the natural history of childhood tuberculosis showed that primary infection, before 2 years of age, frequently progressed to serious disease within the first 12 months without significant prior symptoms [15]. Of the 1,244 cases with tuberculous meningitis or disseminated tuberculosis registered in 2005 and reported to the EuroTB project by 27 countries (European Union member states, western European countries and the Balkan countries), 151 (12%) were in children. Romania reported 72 (48%) of the total 151 cases in children.

Miller and Taylor (1963) [23] observed that among children younger than 1 year of age, with reactive TST, pulmonary lesions developed in 43% and 15-20% had meningitis or miliary disease. EuroTB data revealed that the proportion of children with pulmonary disease in 2004 was 55.3%. This is compared to 68.1% in 2000 and that in 2004, 25% of childhood cases had intrathoracic lymph node disease compared to the overall rate of 2.4%.

Tuberculous meningitis is the most severe form of childhood tuberculosis with mortality or long-term neurological sequelae occurring in almost 50% of cases. In Europe, tuberculous meningitis made up 1.7% of all disease in children aged 0-14 years-old compared to 0.6% of adults cases in 2004 [40]. In Peru, cases of tuberculous meningitis in children aged under 5 years-old decreased from 3.4 per 100,000 in 1992 to 0.8 per 100,000 in 2000 [38]. Approximately 85% of children present tuberculous meningitis with advance (stage II or III) disease, irrespective of their HIV status [45]. Approximately, 45% of HIV-infected children and two-thirds of HIV-uninfected children with tuberculous meningitis have a positive TST (defined as ≥ 5 mm for HIV-infected patients and ≥ 10 mm for HIV-uninfected patients) [45, 46]. Studies have shown that young age and HIV infection are risk factors for more severe, disseminated disease, and have estimated that HIV infection increases the risk of tuberculosis disease by a factor of 20 [47].

3.5. EPIDEMIOLOGY OF DRUG-RESISTANT TUBERCULOSIS

Concerning the specific treatment for tuberculosis, Multidrug-resistant tuberculosis (MDR-TB) is a form of disease that does not respond to the standard treatments regimen using first-line drugs. MDR-TB is defined as resistance to both isoniazid and rifampicin with or without other drugs, and it is present in virtually all countries surveyed by World Health Organization (WHO) and its partners. The WHO estimates that

511,000 new cases of MDR-TB occurred in 2007 with three countries accounting for 56% of all cases globally: China, India and the Russian Federation; about 4.9% of all tuberculosis cases [48]. And of these, 40,000 (6.6%) are estimated to be the Extensively drug-resistant tuberculosis (XDR-TB) [49; 50]. On the other hand, the XDR-TB occurs when resistance to second-line drugs develops. It is extremely difficult to treat and cases have been confirmed in more than 50 countries. WHO's Stop Tuberculosis Strategy aims to reach all patients and achieve the target under the Millennium Development Goals: to reduce by 2015 the prevalence of deaths due to tuberculosis by 50% relative to 1990 and reverse the trend in incidence. The strategy emphasizes the need for proper health systems and the importance of effective primary health care to address the tuberculosis epidemic [1; 2].

Comprehensive studies on resistance to anti-tuberculosis drugs in children are limited (see chapter 2). Drug-resistant tuberculosis in children is usually primary resistance, as children are generally less likely to have been treated previously [39]. In general, the incidence and types of resistant bacilli encountered in children reflect the organisms circulating in the community. A South African study, conducted between 1994 and 1998 in tuberculosis culture-positive children, found 5.6% had isoniazid resistance and 1% had multi-drug resistance [51]. Between 2003 and 2005, it has been shown a similar rate of MDR-TB but a significant increase in isoniazid resistance, from 6,9% to 12,8% reflecting the ongoing transmission of drug-resistant tuberculosis [52]. Also, another study that followed up childhood contacts under 5 years-old living with adults with pulmonary MDR-TB confirmed that 24% had developed disease, whereas 54% were infected within 30 months [53]. These data are alarming as it indicates that resistant organisms are effectively transmitted within the community.

In the UK between 1993 and 1999, the rate of isoniazid resistance in pediatric cases was 6.3%, and of MDR-TB was 0.8%, similar to the rates in adults [54]. At present, there are limited data on the rates of MDR-TB in children in Europe, and thus the best approximation comes from combined adult and pediatric data.

3.6. CONCLUDING REMARKS

Tuberculosis is an important cause of pneumonia worldwide and it could contribute to global childhood mortality. Global estimates of 130,000 deaths due to tuberculosis per year among children have been made. For each 1% annual risk of tuberculosis infection, if active disease is not diagnosed and treated, the estimate mortality rate is 18 per 100,000 infected children aged 0-4 years-old (half of them from tuberculous meningitis), and 9 per 100,000 in those aged 5-14 years-old [36]. Childhood tuberculosis may function as a sensor of the efficacy of tuberculosis-control programmes, but the difficulty in establishing a diagnostic pattern to infant disease impairs the acquisition of reliable statistics of the disease in children. Therefore, WHO research priority guidelines for pediatric tuberculosis have identified the evaluation of new techniques to improve the diagnosis and management of pediatric tuberculosis as an urgent research priority [55].

REFERENCES

[1]   WHO   European   Region.   www   euro   who   int/childhealthenv   2010.   Available   from: www.euro.who.int/childhealthenv (last access Feb. 2010).

[2]   WHO   European   Region.   www   euro   who   int/tuberculosis/TBForum/20071002   2007.   Available   from: www.euro.who.int/tuberculosis/TBForum/20071002 (last access Feb. 2010).

[3]   Ormerod P. The clinical management of the drug-resistant patient. Ann NY Acad Sci 2001; 953: 185-91.

[4]   Murray C, Styblo K, Rouillon A. Tuberculosis in developing countries: burden, intervention and cost. Bull Int Union Tuberc Lung Dis 1990; 65: 6-24.

[5]   Whittaker E, Kampmann B. Perinatal tuberculosis: new challenges in the diagnosis and treatment of tuberculosis in infants and the newborn. Early Hum Dev 2008; 84: 795-9.

[6]   World Health Organization. Guidance for National Tuberculosis Programs on the Management of Tuberculosis in Children. 2006. Report No. 2006.

[7]   Corbett EL, Charalambous S, Moloi VM, *et al.* Human immunodeficiency virus and the prevalence of undiagnosed tuberculosis in African gold miners. Am J Resp Crit Care Med 2004; 170: 673-9.

[8]   Ljghter J, Rigaud M. Diagnosing childhood tuberculosis: traditional and innovative modalities. Curr Probl Pediatr Adolesc Health Care 2009; 39: 61-88.

[9]   Nelson LJ, Wells CD. Global epidemiology of childhood tuberculosis. Int J Tuberc Lung Dis 2004; 8: 636-47.

[10]   Rieder HL. Epidemiology of tuberculosis in children. Ann Nestle 1997; 55: 1-9.

[11]   Lienhardt C, Sillah J, Fielding K, *et al.* Risk factors for tuberculosis infection in children in contact with infectious tuberculosis cases in the Gambia, West Africa. Pediatrics 2003; 111: 608-14.

[12]   Nair SS, Rao GR, Chandrasekhar P. Distribution of tuberculosis infection and disease in clusters of rural households. Indian J Tuberc 1971; 18: 3.

[13]   Kenyon TA, Creek T, Laserson K, *et al.* Risk factors for transmission of *Mycobacterium tuberculosis* from HIV-infected tuberculosis patients, Botswana. Int J Tuberc Lung Dis 2002; 6: 843-50.

[14]   Munoz M, Starke JR. Tuberculosis in children. In: Reichman L.D., Hershfield E.S., editors. Tuberculosis: A Comprehensive International Approach. 2nd ed. Marcel Dekker. New York 2000. pp. 553-86.

[15]   Marais BJ, Gie RP, Schaaf HS, *et al.* The natural history of childhood intra-thoracic tuberculosis: a critical review of literature from the pre-chemotherapy era. Int J Tuberc Lung Dis 2004; 8: 392-402.

[16]   Marais BJ, Gie RP, Obihara CC, Hesseling AC, Schaaf HS, Beyers N. Well-defined symptoms are of value in the diagnosis of childhood pulmonary tuberculosis. Arch Dis Child 2005; 90: 1162-5.

[17]   Newton SM, Brent AJ, Anderson S, Whittaker E, Kampmann B. Paediatric tuberculosis. Lancet Infect Dis 2008; 8: 498-510.

[18]   Marais BJ, Graham SM, Cotton MF, Beyers N. Diagnostic and management challenges for childhood tuberculosis in the era of HIV. J Infect Dis 2007; 196: 76-85.

[19]   Snider DEJ, Rieder HL, Combs D, Bloch AB, Hayden CH, Smith MH. Tuberculosis in children. Pediatr Infect Dis J 1988; 7: 271-8.

[20]   Kessler C, Connolly M, Levy M, Porter J, Rieder HL. Tuberculosis control in refugee populations: a challenge to both relief agencies and national programs. Int J Tuberc Lung Dis 1998; 2: 105-10.

[21]   Cohn KA, Finalle R, O'Hare G, Feris JM, Fernβndez J, Shah SS. Risk factors for intrathoracic tuberculosis in children from economic migrant populations of two Dominican Republic bateyes. Pediatr Infect Dis J 2009; 28(9): 782-6.

[22]   Dye C. Indians leading role in tuberculosis epidemiology and control. Indian J Med Res 2006; 123: 481-4.

[23]   Miller FJW, Taylor MD. Tuberculosis in children. Boston 1963.

[24]   Chintu C, Bhat G, Luo C, *et al.* Seroprevalence of human immunodeficiency virus type 1 infection in Zambian children with tuberculosis. Pediatr Infect Dis J 1993; 12: 499-504.

[25]   Mukadi YD, Wiktor SZ, Coulibaly IM, *et al.* Impact of HIV infection on the development, clinical presentation, and outcome of tuberculosis among children in Abidjan, Cotte d`Ivoire. AIDS 1997; 15: 1151-8.

[26]   Chintu C, Mudenda V, Lucas S, *et al.* Lung diseases at necropsy in African children dying from respiratory illnesses: a descriptive necropsy study. Lancet 2002; 360: 985-90.

[27]   Jeena PM, Pillay P, Pillay T, Coovadia HM. Impact of HIV-1 co-infection on presentation and hospital-related mortality in children with culture proven pulmonary tuberculosis in Durban, South Africa. Int J Tuberc Lung Dis 2002; 6: 672-8.

[28]   Comstock GW, Livesay VT, Woolpert SF. The prognosis of a positive tuberculin reaction in childhood and adolescence. Am J Epidemiol 1974; 99: 131-8.

[29]   Marais BJ, Gie RP, Schaaf HS, Beyers N, Donald PR, Starke JR. Childhood pulmonary tuberculosis: old wisdom and new challenges. Am J Respir Crit Care Med 2006; 173: 1078-99.

[30]   Webb EA, Hesseling AC, Schaaf HS, *et al.* High prevalence of *Mycobacterium tuberculosis* infection and disease in children and adolescents with type 1 diabetes mellitus. Int J Tuberc Lung Dis 2009; 13: 868-74.

[31]   Datta M, Swaminathan S. Global aspects of tuberculosis in children. Paed Respir Rev 2001; 2: 91-6.

[32]   Andresen D. Microbiological diagnostic procedures in respiratory infections: mycobacterial infections. Paediatr Respir Rev 2007; 8: 221-30.

[33]   Zar HJ. Diagnosis of pulmonary tuberculosis in children: what's new? S. Afr. Med J 2007; 97: 983-5.

[34]   Hershfield E. Tuberculosis in children: guidelines for diagnosis, prevention and management (a statement of the scientific committees of the IUATLD). 1991. Report No. 66.

[35]   Rekha B, Swaminathan S. Childhood tuberculosis: global epidemiology and the impact of HIV. Paediatr Resp Rev 2007; 8: 99-106.

[36]   Styblo K. Global scenario. In: Vimlesh S, Kabra SK, editors. Essentials of tuberculosis in children. Jaypee Brothers Medical. New Delhi 2001. pp. 9-18.

[37]   Centers for Disease Control and Prevention. Reported Tuberculosis in the United States, 2001. MMWR; Atlanta: US Department of Health and Human Services; 2002. Report No. 49.

[38]   Carranza MT. Meningoencefalitis tuberculosa (MEC-TB) in menores de 5 anos. Peru. 1993-2000. In: Unión Internacional Contra la Tuberculosis y Enfermedades Respiratorias (UICTER), editor. Programa Nacional de Control de Enfermedades Transmisibles. Tuberculosis en El Peru - Informe 2000. Lima 2001.

[39]   Walls T, Shingadia D. The epidemiology of tuberculosis in Europe. Arch Dis Child 2007; 92(8): 726-9.

[40]   EuroTB. Surveillance of tuberculosis in Europe. Report on tuberculosis cases notified in 2005. Report 2005.

[41]   Balasegaram S, Watson JM, Rose AM, *et al.* A decade of change: tuberculosis in England and Wales 1988-1998. Arch Dis Child 2003; 88: 772-7.

[42]   Eriksson M, Bennet R, Danielsson N. Clinical manifestations and epidemiology of childhood tuberculosis in Stockholm 1976-1995. Scand J Infect Dis 1997; 29: 569-72.

[43]   Rosenfeldt V, Paerregaard A, Fuursted K, Braendholt V, Valerius NH. Childhood tuberculosis in a Scandinavian metropolitan area 1984-93. 1998; 30(1): 53-7.

[44]   Consensus Statement. Formulation of guidelines for diagnosis and treatment of paediatric TB cases under RNTCP. Indian J. Tuberc.; 2004. Report No. 51.

[45]   van der Weert EM, Hartgers NM, Schaaf HS, *et al.* Comparison of diagnostic criteria of tuberculosis meningitis in human immunodeficiency virus-infected and uninfected children. Pediatr Infect Dis J 2006; 25: 65-9.

[46]   Topley JM, Bamber S, Coovadia HM, Corr PD. Tuberculosis meningitis and co-infection with HIV. Ann Trop Paediatr 1998; 18: 261-6.

[47]   Palme IB, Gudetta B, Bruchfeld J, Muhe L, Giesecke J. Impact of human immunodeficiency virus I infection on clinical presentation, treatment outcome and survival in a cohort of Ethiopian children with tuberculosis. Pediatr Infect Dis J 2002; 21: 1053-61.

[48]   World Health Organization. Global Tuberculosis control: epidemiology, strategy, financing report. 2009. Report No. 2009.

[49]   Wells CD, Cegielski JP, Nelson LJ, *et al.* HIV infection and multidrug-resistant tuberculosis: the perfect storm. J Infect Dis 2007; 196: 86-107.

[50]   Kliiman K, Altraja AS. Predictors of extensively drug resistant pulmonary tuberculosis. Ann Intern Med 2009; 150: 766-75.

[51]   Schaaf HS, Gie RP, Beyers N, Sirgel FA, de Klerk PJ, Donald PR. Primary drug-resistant tuberculosis in children. Int J Tuberc Lung Dis 2000; 4: 1149-55.

[52]   Schaaf HS, Marias BJ, Hesseling AC, Gie RP, Beyers N, Donald PR. Childhood drug resistant tuberculosis in the western Cape province of South Africa. Acta Paediatr 2006; 95: 523-8.

[53]   Schaaf HS, Gie RP, Kennedy M, Beyers N, Hesseling PB, Donald PR. Evaluation of young children in contact with adult multidrug-resistant pulmonary tuberculosis: a 30-month follow-up. Pediatrics 2002; 109: 765-71.

[54]   Djuretic T, Herbert J, Drobniewski F, *et al.* Antibiotic resistant tuberculosis in the United Kingdom 1993-1999. Thorax 2002; 57: 477-82.

[55]   World Health Organization. A research agenda for childhood tuberculosis. 2007. Report No. 2007.

CHAPTER 4

Immune Responses for Tuberculosis in the Infected Infant

Dilvani O. Santos[1],* and Paulo R.Z. Antas[2]

[1]*Laboratório de Biopatógenos e Ativação Celular, Departamento de Biologia Celular e Molecular, Instituto de Biologia, Universidade Federal Fluminense, Av. Barros-Terra s/n Valonguinho, zip: 24001-970, Niterói, Rio de Janeiro, Brazil and* [2]*Laboratório de Imunologia Clínica, Fiocruz, Av. Brasil, # 4365; zip: 21045-900, Rio de Janeiro, Brazil*

Abstract: It is estimated that the lifetime risk of developing active disease after infection with *Mycobacterium tuberculosis* in childhood is about 10%. Therefore, the human immune response to *M. tuberculosis* infection prevents the development of illness in most people. Tuberculosis is contagious and spreads through the air. Bacilli can subsequently enter the blood stream where they spread hematogenously throughout the body. If not treated, each person with active tuberculosis disease can infect on average 10 to 15 people per year. The factors that allow for progression to active disease among infected persons are not fully understood, however, they are likely immunologic, based on the increased rates of disease in persons with varying forms of immune response. The source of infection for most children is an infectious adult in a closed environment. This exposure leads to the development of a primary lesion in the lung witch spreads to the regional lymph nodes. In the majority of cases, the resultant cell-mediated immunity controls the disease at this stage. Risk of disease progression is higher in the very young (< 3 years-old) and in immune compromised children. However, children with tuberculosis differ from adults in their immunological and pathophysiological response in ways that may have important implications for the prevention, diagnosis and treatment of this disease in the pediatric population.

Keywords: Tuberculosis, Immune Response, Childhood, BCG.

4.1. BACKGROUND

The protection against *Mycobacterium tuberculosis* requires a link between the innate and adaptive immune system. Nevertheless, tuberculosis is a major cause of mortality worldwide because the tubercle bacilli is exceptionally successful and has infected a third of the world population [1]. Despite the introduction of the Bacille Calmette Guérin (BCG) vaccination in the first half of the 20th century and the availability of efficient anti-tuberculosis therapy since the 1960s, about 2 million of deaths occur annually [2]. The main reasons for the persistence of this ancient disease have been already summarized (see chapter 3), but those factors leading to immunological deficits play a key role. In addition, the percentage of drug-resistant bacilli is increasing [3; 4]. Another considerable issue is the unsatisfying efficacy of BCG that prevents severe disease in childhood, but not the most common pulmonary infection of adults [5, 6]. For this reason, several newly developed candidate vaccines have reached the level of clinical trials [7]. Another strategy follows the idea that secreted mycobacterial immunedominant antigens will induce protective memory T lymphocytes when given as fusion proteins [8-10], or if expressed in a modified vaccinia virus Ankara [11]. Current approaches include DNA vaccines, genetically modified viable mycobacteria, and subunit vaccines [12]. To cover this particular subject, outstanding reviews are presently accessible elsewhere for consulting. Traditionally, the search for immunogenic mycobacterial antigens, to be included in a subunit vaccine, has focused on classical protein antigens-stimulating CD4 T cells [13]. More recently, the translation of basic research into vaccine design prompted the search for unconventional antigens that stimulate T cells or CD1-restricted T cells [14, 15]. Cells responding to non-protein antigens are likely to be important in protection against tuberculosis because they produce Th1 cytokines, lyse *M. tuberculosis*-infected cells, and directly kill the intracellular pathogen *via* the peptide granulysin [15].

*Address correspondence to Dilvani O. Santos: Laboratório de Biopatógenos e Ativação Celular, Departamento de Biologia Celular e Molecular, Instituto de Biologia, Universidade Federal Fluminense, Av. Barros-Terra s/n Valonguinho, zip: 24001-970, Niterói, Rio de Janeiro, Brazil; Tel: +55 21 2629-2290 / +55 21 2629-2294; E-mail: santosdilvani@gmail.com

During the 20th century, major advances occurred in the diagnosis and treatment of tuberculosis. Detection of infection became possible with the tuberculin skin test (TST), and diagnosis of disease was enhanced with the use of chest X-ray. The TST (also known as Mantoux, Pirquet or PPD test) is an approach used to determine if someone has developed an immune response against *M. tuberculosis*. This response can occur if someone either: currently has tuberculosis, was exposed to it in the past, or has received the BCG vaccine against tuberculosis (which is not performed in the U.S.A.).

The TST is based on the fact that infection with *M. tuberculosis* produces a delayed-type hypersensitivity skin reaction to certain components of the bacilli. The components of the organism are contained in extracts of culture filtrates and are the core elements of the classic, "old" tuberculin. This tuberculin crude material, purified protein derivative (PPD), is used for skin testing in order to detect tuberculosis. Reaction in the skin to tuberculin compounds begins when T cells, which have been sensitized by prior infection, are recruited by the immune system to the skin site where they release cytokines and chemokines. These molecules induce induration, (a hard, raised area with clearly defined margins at and around the injection site), through local vasodilatation, (expansion of the diameter of blood vessels), leading to edema, fibrin deposition, and recruitment of other types of inflammatory cells to the area (more details at chapter 6).

An incubation period from 2 to 12 weeks is usually necessary, after exposure to the tubercle bacilli, in order to the TST become positive. Also, the diagnosis of latent *M. tuberculosis* infection with a TST in children is complicated by the potential influence of prior exposure to BCG vaccination.

4.2. GENERATION OF IMMUNE RESPONSES

4.2.1. The Role Played by Myeloid Lineage Cells

The immune response against tuberculosis plays an essential role in the outcome of *M. tuberculosis* infection. Tuberculosis is contagious and spreads through the air [16]. In a TST-negative infant, subsequent to an aerosol infection with a few *M. tuberculosis* bacilli, a primary focus of infection is locally established which is primarily, initially, featured by densely intracellular multiplication of the organism. At earlier stages, polymorphonuclear phagocytes, such as neutrophils are also attracted. Neutrophils are among the earliest cells recruited into sites where harmful agents enter the body. The function of neutrophils goes beyond their microbicidal ability, since these cells are thought to contribute to the control of infection through the production of chemokines and the induction of granuloma formation [17]. They also have well-characterized microbicidal mechanisms, such as those dependent on oxygen and which can be transferred to infected macrophages [18]: Although the role played by these cells in tuberculosis infection is controversial.

However, the bacilli has predilection to proliferate within the alveolar macrophages, particularly in the lower lobes of the lung maybe due to aerodynamical reasons [19]. Actually, it appears that *M. tuberculosis* has adapted to employ any of several cellular molecules plentifully present on the surface of macrophages, such as the complement CR3 and CR4, and the Fc receptors [20], fibronectin receptors [21], the mannose receptor [22], surfactant protein [23], CD14 [24], and CD43 [25]. The interaction of bacilli with Fc receptors increases the production of those microbicidal mechanisms dependent on oxygen and allows the fusion of the bacteria-containing phagosomes with lysosomes [26]. Conversely, interaction of bacilli with CR3 prevents the respiratory burst [27] and blocks the maturation of phagosomes harboring the bacilli, thus preventing fusion with lysosomes [28]. Engagement of *M. tuberculosis* surface components with members of the Toll-like receptor (TLR)-2 [29] and TLR-4 [30] has been described, as the 19-kDa lipoprotein and lipoarabinomanann (LAM) activate macrophages through TLR-2, promoting the production of Interleukin-12 (IL-12) and inducible nitric oxide synthase enzyme [29]. Some authors use to refer to macrophage as a paradigmatic cell with regard to *M. tuberculosis* infection [31]. However, the current consensus is that alveolar macrophage has long been considered the first cell population to interact with the tubercle bacilli, and thus play an essential role in the elimination of particles that enter the organism through the airways. Once the bacteria enter the macrophage, they generally locate themselves in the mycobacterial phagosome; whereas in contrast to normal phagocytosis, during which the phagosomal content is degraded upon fusion with lysosomes, the mycobacteria block this process [26, 32]. This inhibition may be reverted by interferon-gamma (IFN-γ) and tumor necrosis factor (TNF), which also stimulate those microbicidal mechanisms [33]; but this key aspect during the infection has not been fully explained, though it is known that hydrogen peroxide produced by macrophages activated by cytokines has mycobactericidal activity [34]. Also, it has been found that *M. tuberculosis* presents molecules, such as LAM and phenolic glycolipid 1, which work as oxygen radical scavenger molecules [33, 35].

Other cell populations, such as dendritic cells (DC), are clearly involved in the protective immune response against *M. tuberculosis* infection. Thus, DC induce maturation of T cells towards a Th1 profile by secreting cytokines, such as IL-12, IL-18, IL-23, and probably IFN-α and β, but not IFN-γ [36-39]. Th1 cells expand in response to mycobacteria antigens presented by DC in the lymphoid tissues and migrate toward infection sites, such as the lung parenchyma, where they release IFN-γ, thus activating local macrophages that control bacilli replication [40]. Some facts about DC are listed below:

- DC recognize and capture antigens by endocytosis using both Fcγ and Fcε receptors, and dendritic cell-specific intercellular-adhesion-molecule-grabbing non-integrin (DC-SIGN) which ligand is LAM [41-43].

- DC process antigens and present them in the context of major histocompatibility complex (MHC) and CD1-like molecules [44, 45].

- DC express both TLR2 and TLR4 [38, 46].

- Interactions LAM and DC-SIGN induce IL-10 production [42], while interactions 19 kDa lipoprotein and TLR-2 induce IL-12, TNF, and IL-6 productions [47-49].

- During maturation, DC not only increase the MHC class I and II synthesis, but also the expression of co-stimulatory molecules, such as CD80 and CD86 [50], and the production of IL-12 [51].

4.2.2. The Role Played by Lymphoid Lineage Cells

Also lymphocytes use to play a very important role in the initial steps and, more importantly, during the development of adaptive immune response against *M. tuberculosis* infections. Those cells belonging to lymphoid lineage are:

- Natural killer (NK) cells, which their main function has been associated with the development of cytotoxicity to infected macrophages and they are among the first cell populations to secrete IFN-γ, and also to express both activation and maturation markers during the initiation of immune response;

- Natural killer T (NKT) cells, which are CD1d-restricted and binds to the invariant Vα24 TCR, and their main functions include IFN-γ secretion, proliferation, cytotoxicity, and direct anti-antimicrobial activity;

- Gamma-delta T cells, which are a subset of T lymphocytes believed to proliferate only in response to non-protein antigens [52], and also found in early lesions thought to react to infected macrophages through cytotoxicity mechanism and IL-17 and IFN-γ productions [53];

- CD4+ and CD8+ T cells, the main arm of specific immune response that will perform the key features toward a protective Th1 phenotype (see below).

The cells involved in this initial and crucial step of the immune response in tuberculosis are listed bellow:

Innate immune response against *M. tuberculosis*

Myeloid lineage	Lymphoid lineage
Polymorphonuclear neutrophils	*Natural killer cells*
Monocytes/Macrophages	*Natural killer T cells*
Dendritic cells	*Gamma/delta T cells*

Another important mechanism of immunity against *M. tuberculosis* infection involves the specific, adaptive immune response. Also relevant, there are very few discrepancies that have been revealed between adults and children regarding this issue. Therefore, this topic will not be fully described in this chapter since it has been already extensively reviewed in excellent text books currently available in an open access mode. It should, however, be considered that the two main arms of adaptive immunity that play distinct and specific roles in *M. tuberculosis* infection are denoted below:

Acquired immune response against *M. tuberculosis*

Humoral immune response	Main features are antibody secretion, T-cell dependent, not fully protective.
Cellular immune response	Main features are key components of a Th1-induced profile orchestrated by CD4+ and CD8+ T cells, and are very protective.

Shortly after establishment of a focus of *M. tuberculosis* infection in the lung, with the recruitment of blood mononuclear cells, the process of *M. tuberculosis* priming of CD4 and CD8 T lymphocytes leading to adaptive immune response is promptly initiated. However time is an issue, and for protective immunity to become adequately vigorous to contain the *M. tuberculosis* growth requires up to 3 weeks. Meanwhile, uncontrolled intracellular replication continues which, eventually, may culminate in the rupture of infected phagocytes and spread the infection to surrounding cells. Also, phagocyte ruptures allow the initiation of both extracellular growth and tissue damage, leading to caseation necrosis, and finally ending in dangerous spread of bacilli in the outside air. Here resides the very risky scenario regarding tuberculosis dissemination, particularly when the pediatric population is in close contact to an adult index case of active disease. As *M. tuberculosis* growth expands, hematogenous spread allows the seeding of bacilli in both upper lobes of the lung and extrapulmonary sites. It should be mentioned that the BCG vaccine in children plays a very critical role to avoid the latter. Finally, with the development of specific, adaptive host cell-mediated immune response, mycobacterial replication is eventually controlled (see chapter 2).

Protective immunity involves the host's capacity to produce T cell cytokines. With this regard, the production and activity of cytokines that are crucial for the development of Th1 immune responses are critical to the final containment of infection. However, the ability of *M. tuberculosis* to persist in a dormant state within host tissues is not yet fully understood, but most probably relies on the capacity of the pathogen to switch its metabolism from a rapid to a slow anaerobic growth [54]. The average rate for infants to switch the structure of the initial granulomatous response induced by *M. tuberculosis* for initiation or termination of dormancy is still unclear. However, conditions that weaken cell-mediated immunity increase the chance of terminating the latent state of infection and development of active tuberculosis disease. The factors that are important in the maintenance of protective immunity against *M. tuberculosis* infection after primary infection are also not known. It is possible that the sustenance of successful immunological surveillance after *M. tuberculosis* infection is contingent on a dynamic interaction in situ within the granuloma, which is permissive to the continuous sensitization of *M. tuberculosis*-reactive T cells, that may, in turn, be dependent upon the low grade replication of a few remaining bacilli. Under this scenario, the coincidence of the breakdown of the immune system (such as an eventual HIV infection), with the low grade periodic mycobacterial replication within "healed" *M. tuberculosis*-infected foci, is likely to be conducive to initiation of the process of reactivation and exponential growth of *M. tuberculosis*. With this regard, again, the capacity of *M. tuberculosis* to induce cytokines that are suppressive to T cell function, deactivate macrophages and damage the tissues is noteworthy.

In addition to the above considerations, the knowledge about T lymphocyte responses in human newborns is still limited. *In vitro* studies on cord blood, mononuclear cells have shown that newborn lymphocytes have a defective IFNγ production in response to mitogens [55; 56].

The Th1-type immune response induced by BCG in newborns is likely to be dependent on the activation of antigen presenting cells. As already denoted, DC are the antigen presenting cells involved in the initiation of primary immune responses. Mycobacteria (including BCG) infect DC and markedly increase their ability to present antigens to T cells [57; 58]. Interestingly, in the presence of IL-12 and optimal co-stimulatory signals, human newborn T lymphocytes promptly differentiate into Th1 cells [59]. Although protective immunity against mycobacterial infections in neonates is not fully understood, a Th1-type immune response is known to be required [60].

Another interesting issue to be considered is the natural history of tuberculosis disease descriptions that do not include the influence of HIV. However, recent disease reports in HIV-infected children confirm that those with significant lack of immunity illustrate poor disease containment, similar to that seen in children under 2 years-old who are immune immature. The definition of relevant disease in immune-compromised children is therefore similar to that in those under 2 years-old and includes any infection, recent or past, primary or re-infection [61-66].

As already mentioned, *M. tuberculosis* is largely controlled by the cellular arm of immunity. A latent tuberculosis infection is characterized by a strong cellular immune response in the absence of detectable bacterial load. In immunocompetent individuals, this persisting immunity is thought to keep bacterial replication to below detectable levels. However, in other forms of decreased immune response, as in iatrogenic immunosuppression in transplant recipients, it accounts for a progressive impairment in cellular immunity that may contribute to an increased incidence of reactivation from latent tuberculosis infection to active disease. In addition, a higher rate of primary tuberculosis infections due to regular visits of dialysis units, or also after organ transplants, may further increase the risk for tuberculosis infectious complications in transient immunecompromised patients [67].

Concerning the effectiveness of tuberculosis diagnosis, the whole-blood assay reveals a high prevalence of latent tuberculosis infection in renal transplant recipients. It may represent a valuable alternative to tuberculin skin testing as the result is not adversely affected by immunesuppression (see chapter 6). Moreover, reactivity towards more specific *M. tuberculosis* antigens allows the distinction of a latent infection from BCG-induced reactivity [68]. The assay is well-suited for use in screening programmes and may facilitate the management of tuberculosis infection in immunocompromised individuals [68].

4.3. CONCLUDING REMARKS

A substantial amount of clinical experience indicates that host cell immunity plays an important role in the host-pathogen interactions occurring in infants exposed to *M. tuberculosis*. Furthermore, the neonatal BCG vaccination should represent one of the first infectious challenges during life - it could have a strong effect on the development of immune system of the infant. Understanding the components of this host response, mainly in infants, at a basic level is likely to lead to a better understanding of the pathogenesis of tuberculosis in humans and result in improved and novel approaches for prevention and management of this disease: Which, among adults, remains the leading cause of death by a single pathogen in the world today.

REFERENCES

[1]   World Health Organization. Global Tuberculosis control: epidemiology, strategy, financing report. 2009. Report No. 2009.

[2]   World Health Organization. Global Tuberculosis Control. 2007. Report No. 2007.

[3]   Centers for Disease Control and Prevention. Emergence of *Mycobacterium tuberculosis* with extensive resistance to second line drugs, 2000-2004. MMWR; 2006. Report No. 55.

[4]   Friedland G. Tuberculosis,drug resistance,and HIV/AIDS: a triple threat. Curr Infect Dis Rep 2007; 9: 252-61.

[5]   Brewer TF. Preventing tuberculosis with Bacillus Calmette-Guerin vaccine: a meta-analysis of the literature. Clin Infect Dis 2000; 31: 64-7.

[6]   Trunz BB, Fine P, Dye C. Effect of BCG vaccination on childhood tuberculous meningitis and miliary tuberculosis worldwide: a meta-analysis and assessment of cost-effectiveness. Lancet 2006; 367: 1173-80.

[7]   Skeiky YA, Sadoff JC. Advances in tuberculosis vaccine strategies. Nat Rev Microbiol 2006; 4(6): 469-76.

[8]   Olsen AW, Williams A, Okkels LM, Hatch G, Andersen P. Protective effect of a tuberculosis subunit vaccine based on a fusion of antigen 85B and ESAT-6 in the aerosol guinea pig model. Infect Immun 2004; 72: 6148-50.

[9]   Brandt L, Skeiky YA, Alderson MR, *et al.* The protective effect of the *Mycobacterium bovis* BCG vaccine is increased by coadministration with the *Mycobacterium tuberculosis* 72-kilodalton fusion polyprotein Mtb72F in *M. tuberculosis*-infected guinea pigs. Infect Immun 2004; 72: 6622-32.

[10]   Langermans JA, Doherty TM, Vervenne RA, *et al.* Protection of macaques against *Mycobacterium tuberculosis* infection by a subunit vaccine based on a fusion protein of antigen 85B and ESAT-6. Vaccine 2005; 23: 2740-50.

[11]   McShane H, Pathan AA, Sander CR, *et al.* Recombinant modified vaccinia virus Ankara expressing antigen 85A boosts BCG-primed and naturally acquired antimycobacterial immunity in humans. Nat Med 2004; 10(11): 1240-4.

[12]   Kaufmann SH, McMichael AJ. Annulling a dangerous liaison: vaccination strategies against AIDS and tuberculosis. Nat Med 2005; 11: S33-S44.

[13]   Boom WH, Canaday DH, Fulton SA, Gehring AJ, Rojas RE, Torres M. Human immunity to *M. tuberculosis*: T cell subsets and antigen processing. Tuberculosis 2003; 83: 98-106.

[14]   Kaufmann SH. Recent findings in immunology give tuberculosis vaccines a new boost. Trends Immunol 2005; 26: 660-7.

[15]   Behar SM, Porcelli SA. CD1-restricted T cells in host defense to infectious diseases. Curr Top Microbiol Immunol 2007; 314: 215-50.

[16]   Stead WW. Management of health care workers after inadvertent exposure to tuberculosis: a guide for the use of preventive therapy. Ann Intern Med 1995; 122: 906-12.

[17]   Riedel DD, Kaufmann SH. Chemokine secretion by human polymorphonuclear granulocytes after stimulation with *Mycobacterium tuberculosis* and lipoarabinomannan. Infect Immun 1997; 65: 4620-3.

[18]   Tan BH, Meinken C, Bastian M, *et al.* Macrophages acquire neutrophil granules for antimicrobial activity against intracellular pathogens. J Immunol 2006; 177: 1864-71.

[19]   Hirsch CS, Ellner JJ, Russell DG, Rich EA. Complement receptor mediated uptake and tumor necrosis alpha-mediated growth inhibition of *Mycobacterium tuberculosis* by human alveolar macrophages. J Immunol 1994; 152: 743-9.

[20]   Schlesinger LS, Bellinger-Kawahara CG, Payne NR, Horowitz MA. Phagocytosis of *Mycobacterium tuberculosis* is mediated by human monocyte complement receptors and complement component C3. J Immunol 1990; 144: 2771-80.

[21]   Ratliff TL, McGarr JA, Abou-Zeid C, *et al.* Attachment of mycobacteria to fibronectin-coated surfaces. J Gen Microbiol 1988; 134: 1307-13.

[22]   Schlesinger LS. Macrophage phagocytosis of virulent but not attenuated strains of *Mycobacterium tuberculosis* is mediated by mannose receptors in addition to complement receptors. J Immunol 1993; 150: 2920-30.

[23]   Zimmerli S, Edwards S, Ernst JD. Selective receptor blockade during phagocytosis does not alter the survival and growth of *Mycobacterium tuberculosis* in human macrophages. Am J Respir Cell Mol Biol 1996; 15: 760-70.

[24]   Peterson PK, Gekker G, Hu S, *et al.* CD14 receptor-mediated uptake of nonopsonized *Mycobacterium tuberculosis* by human microglia. Infect Immun 1995; 63: 1598-602.

[25]   Randhawa AK, Ziltener HJ, Merzaban JS, Stokes RW. CD43 is required for optimal growth inhibition of *Mycobacterium tuberculosis* in macrophages and in mice. J Immunol 2005; 175: 1805-12.

[26]   Armstrong JA, Hart PD. Phagosome-lysosome interactions in cultured macrophages infected with virulent tubercle bacilli: Reversal of the usual nonfusion pattern and observations on bacterial survival. J Exp Med 1975; 142: 1-16.

[27]   Le Cabec V, Cols C, Maridonneau-Parini I. Nonopsonic phagocytosis of zymosan and *Mycobacterium kansasii* by CR3 (CD11b/CD18) involves distinct molecular determinants and is or is not coupled with NADPH oxidase activation. Infect Immun 2000; 68: 4736-45.

[28] Sturgill-Koszycki S, Schlesinger PH, Chakraborty P, Haddix PL, Collins HL, Fok AK, *et al.* Lack of acidification in Mycobacterium phagosomes produced by exclusion of the vesicular proton-ATPase. Science 1994 Feb 4; 263(5147): 678-81.

[29] Brightbill HD, Libraty DH, Krutzik SR, *et al.* Host defense mechanisms triggered by microbial lipoproteins through toll-like receptors. Science 1999; 285: 732-6.

[30] Jiang W, Swiggard WJ, Heufler C, *et al.* The receptor DEC-205 expressed by dendritic cells and thymic epithelial cells is involved in antigen processing. Nature 1995; 375: 151-5.

[31] Tuberculosis 2007. Available from: http: //www tuberculosistextbook com/index htm 2007 (last access Feb. 2010).

[32] Armstrong JA, Hart PD. Response of cultured macrophages to *Mycobacterium tuberculosis* with observations on fusion of lysosomes with phagosomes. J Exp Med 1971; 134: 713-40.

[33] Chan X, Xing Y, Magliozzo RS, Bloom BR. Killing of virulent *Mycobacterium tuberculosis* by reactive nitrogen intermediates produced by activated macrophages. J Exp Med 1992; 175: 1111-22.

[34] Walker L, Lowrie DB. Killing of *Mycobacterium microti* by immunologically activated macrophages. Nature 1981; 293: 69-71.

[35] Chan J, Fan XD, Hunter SW, Brennan PJ, Bloom BR. Lipoarabinomannan,a possible virulence factor involved in persistence of *Mycobacterium tuberculosis* within macrophages. Infect Immun 1991; 59: 1755-61.

[36] Thurnher M, Ramoner R, Gastl G, *et al.* Bacillus Calmette-Guerin mycobacteria stimulate human blood dendritic cells. Int J Cancer 1997; 70: 128-34.

[37] Kalinski P, Schuitemaker.J.H., Hilkens CM, Wierenga EA, Kapsenberg ML. Final maturation of dendritic cells is associated with impaired responsiveness to IFN-gamma and to bacterial IL-12 inducers: decreased ability of mature dendritic cells to produce IL-12 during the interaction with Th cells. J Immunol 1999; 162: 3231-6.

[38] Kadowaki N, Ho S, Antonenko S, *et al.* Subsets of human dendritic cell precursors express different toll-like receptors and respond to different microbial antigens. J Exp Med 2001; 194: 863-9.

[39] Wozniak TM, Ryan AA, Triccas JA, Britton WJ. Plasmid interleukin-23 (IL-23),but not plasmid IL-27, enhances the protective efficacy of a DNA vaccine against *Mycobacterium tuberculosis* infection. Infect Immun 2006; 74: 557-65.

[40] Humphreys IR, Stewart GR, Turner DJ, *et al.* A role for dendritic cells in the dissemination of mycobacterial infection. Microbes Infect 2006; 8: 1339-46.

[41] Figdor CG, van Kooyk Y, Adema GJ. C-type lectin receptors on dendritic cells and Langerhans cells. Nat Rev Immunol 2002; 2: 77-84.

[42] Geijtenbeek TB, van Vliet SJ, Koppel EA, *et al.* Mycobacteria target DC-SIGN to suppress dendritic cell function. J Exp Med 2003; 197: 7-17.

[43] Tailleux L, Schwartz O, Herrmann JL, *et al.* DC-SIGN is the major *Mycobacterium tuberculosis* receptor on human dendritic cells. J Exp Med 2003 Jan 6; 197(1): 121-7.

[44] Banchereau J, Steinman RM. Dendritic cells and the control of immunity. Nature 1998; 392: 245-52.

[45] Gumperz JE, Brenner MB. CD1-specific T cells in microbial immunity. Curr Opin Immunol 2001; 13: 471-8.

[46] Jarrossay D, Napolitani G, Colonna M, Sallusto F, Lanzavecchia A. Specialization and complementarity in microbial molecule recognition by human myeloid and plasmacytoid dendritic cells. Eur J Immunol 2001; 31: 3388-93.

[47] Means TK, Wang S, Lien E, Yoshimura A, Golenbock DT, Fenton MJ. Human toll-like receptors mediate cellular activation by Mycobacterium tuberculosis. J Immunol 1999; 163: 3920-7.

[48] Underhill DM, Ozinsky A, Smith KD, Aderem A. Toll-like receptor-2 mediates mycobacteria-induced proinflammatory signaling in macrophages. Proc Natl Acad Sci USA 1999; 96: 14459-63.

[49] Means TK, Jones BW, Schromm AB, *et al.* Differential effects of a Toll-like receptor antagonist on *Mycobacterium tuberculosis*-induced macrophage responses. J Immunol 2001; 166: 4074-82.

[50] Turley SJ, Inaba K, Garrett WS, *et al.* Transport of peptide-MHC class II complexes in developing dendritic cells. Science 2000; 288: 522-7.

[51] Steinman RM. Dendritic cells and the control of immunity: enhancing the efficiency of antigen presentation. Mt Sinai J Med 2001; 68: 160-6.

[52] Schoel B, Sprenger S, Kaufmann SH. Phosphate is essential for stimulation of V gamma 9 V delta 2 T lymphocytes by mycobacterial low molecular weight ligand. Eur J Immunol 1994; 24: 1886-92.

[53] Ferrick DA, Schrenzel MD, Mulvania T, Hsieh B, Ferlin WG, Lepper H. Differential production of interferon-gamma and interleukin-4 in response to Th1- and Th2-stimulating pathogens by gamma delta T cells *in vivo.* Nature 1995; 373: 255-7.

[54] Wayne LG, Hayes LG. An *in vitro* model for sequential study of shiftdown of *Mycobacterium tuberculosis* through two stages of nonreplicating persistence. Infect Immun 1996; 64: 2062-9.

[55] Wilson CB, Westall J, Johnston L, Lewis DB, Dower SK, Alpert AR. Decreased production of interferon-gamma by human neonatal cells: Intrinsic and regulatory deficiencies. J Clin Invest 1986; 77: 860-7.

[56] Roncarolo MG, Bigler M, Ciuti E, Martino S, Tovo PA. Immune responses by cord blood cells. Blood cells 1994; 20: 573-85.

[57] Inaba K, Inaba M, Naito M, Steinman RM. Dendritic cell progenitors phagocytose particulates including Bacillus Calmette-Guerin organisms, and sensitize mice to mycobacterial antigens *in vivo*. J Exp Med 1993; 178: 479-88.

[58] Henderson RA, Watkins SC, Flynn JL. Activation of human dendritic cells following infection with *Mycobacterium tuberculosis*. J Immunol 1997 Jul 15; 159(2): 635-43.

[59] Ohshima Y, Delespesse G. T cell-derived IL-4 and dendritic cell-derived IL-12 regulate the lymphokine-producing phenotype of alloantigen-primed naive human CD4 T cells. J Immunol 1997; 158: 629-36.

[60] Marchant A, Goetghebuer T, Ota MO, *et al.* Newborns develop a Th1-type immune response to *Mycobacterium bovis* bacillus Calmette-Guerin vaccination. J Immunol 1999 Aug 15; 163(4): 2249-55.

[61] Chan SP, Birnbaum J, Rao M, Steiner P. Clinical manifestations and outcome of tuberculosis in children with acquired immune deficiency syndrome. Pediatr Infect Dis J 1996; 15: 443-7.

[62] Mukadi YD, Wiktor SZ, Coulibaly IM, *et al.* Impact of HIV infection on the development, clinical presentation, and outcome of tuberculosis among children in Abidjan, Cotte d'Ivoire. AIDS 1997; 15: 1151-8.

[63] Madhi SA, Huebner RE, Doedens L, Aduc T, Wesley D, Cooper PA. HIV-1 co-infection in children hospitalised with tuberculosis in South Africa. Int J Tuberc Lung Dis 2000; 4(5): 448-54.

[64] Graham SM, Coulter JB, Gilks CF. Pulmonary disease in HIV-infected African children. Int J Tuberc Lung Dis 2001; 5: 12-23.

[65] Palme IB, Gudetta B, Bruchfeld J, Muhe L, Giesecke J. Impact of human immunodeficiency virus I infection on clinical presentation, treatment outcome and survival in a cohort of Ethiopian children with tuberculosis. Pediatr Infect Dis J 2002; 21: 1053-61.

[66] Marais BJ, Gie RP, Schaaf HS, *et al.* The natural history of childhood intra-thoracic tuberculosis: a critical review of literature from the pre-chemotherapy era. Int J Tuberc Lung Dis 2004; 8: 392-402.

[67] Spence RK, Dafoe DC, Rabin G, *et al.* Mycobacterial infections in renal allograft recipients. Arch Surg 1983; 118: 356-9.

[68] Sester U, Junker H, Hodapp T, *et al.* Improved efficiency in detecting cellular immunity towards *M. tuberculosis* in patients receiving immunosuppressive drug therapy. Nephrol Dial Transplant 2006; 21(11): 3258-68.

CHAPTER 5

Classical Diagnosis of Tuberculosis

Roberta O. Pinheiro[1,*] and Paulo R.Z. Antas[2]

[1]Leprosy Laboratory, Fiocruz, Av. Brasil, # 4365; zip: 21045-900, Rio de Janeiro, Brazil and [2]Laboratório de Imunologia Clínica, Fiocruz, Av. Brasil, # 4365; zip: 21045-900, Rio de Janeiro, Brazil

Abstract: The diagnosis of children tuberculosis involves the clinical, epidemiology and image methods, as well as the results of a tuberculin skin test. Tuberculosis can mimic many common childhood diseases, including pneumonia, generalized bacterial and viral infections, malnutrition and HIV. The main impediment to the accurate diagnosis of active tuberculosis is the paucibacillary nature of the disease in children. Although the diagnosis of tuberculosis disease in adults is mainly bacteriologic, in children it is usually epidemiologic and, therefore, indirect. In the absence of accurate diagnostic tools for tuberculosis in children, both underdiagnosis and overdiagnosis are common. The overdiagnosis is exacerbated in areas with a high prevalence of HIV and tuberculosis because both share many clinical features, often making it impossible to exclude tuberculosis in HIV-infected children. Many adults who develop infectious reactivation of tuberculosis acquired the infection during childhood. Given the effectiveness of isoniazid preventive therapy to stop progression of active tuberculosis, accurate diagnosis and treatment of *M. tuberculosis* infection in children would reduce many cases of contagious, adult, tuberculosis in the future.

Keywords: Children Tuberculosis, Clinical Diagnosis, Radiological Diagnosis, Bacteriological Diagnosis, Immunological and Biochemical Diagnosis.

5.1. CLINICAL DIAGNOSIS

Many cases of primary tuberculosis infection in children are asymptomatic, self-healing, and remain completely unnoticed. The diagnosis of childhood tuberculosis is further complicated by the absence of a practical gold standard. Given this situation, the diagnosis of childhood tuberculosis is often made solely on the key clinical features of chronic symptoms, physical signs, a possible tuberculin skin test (TST) reaction, and/or a chest X-ray suggestive of disease [1].

In some countries score charts are used to tuberculosis diagnosis, although they have rarely been evaluated against a gold standard. The diagnostic scoring system used by the Brazilian Ministry of Health is among the diagnostic systems assessed [2]. It has been validated and presents a good balance between sensitivity and specificity (89% and 87%, respectively), making it useful in areas where tuberculosis and HIV co-infection is low (Table **1**). A review of existing scoring systems found that 5 out of 17 methods had been adapted for use in HIV-infected children, while only one had been specially developed for use in such population [3]. The World Health Organization (WHO) recommends that score charts should therefore be used as screening tools and not as the means of making a firm diagnosis [4].

Table 1. Score System for Diagnosis of Sputum-Negative Children and Adolescents.

BCG* vaccination and Tuberculin Skin Test (TST)	Score
BCG > 2 years or no TST ≥ 10 mm	+15
BCG < 2 years or no TST ≥ 15 mm	+15
BCG yes/no TST 5 mm to 9 mm	+5
BCG yes/no TST ≤ 5 mm	0

*Address correspondence to Roberta O. Pinheiro:** Leprosy Laboratory, Fiocruz, Av. Brasil, # 4365; zip: 21045-900, Rio de Janeiro, Brazil; Fax: +55 21 2270-9997, E-mail: rolmo@ioc.fiocruz.br

Paulo Renato Zuquim Antas, Dilvani Oliveira Santos, Roberta Olmo Pinheiro and Theolis Barbosa (Eds)

Table 1. cont....

Clinical manifestations	Score
Fever or cough, lost energy, sputum, lost weight, night sweats > 2 weeks	+15
No symptoms or symptoms < 2 weeks	0
Respiratory infection improving with or without antibioticotherapy for common bacteria	-10

Thoracic/chest X-ray	Score
Enlarged hilum or military pattern / Exsudate or patch shadow (with or without cavitation) unaltered > 2 weeks or worst with antibioticotherapy for common bacteria.	+15
Exsudate or patch shadow (with or without cavitation) < 2 weeks	+5
Normal	-5

Nutritional status	Score
Severe malnutrition	+5
Eutrophic or no severe malnutrition	0

Contact with tubercle adult	Score
Close, <2 years	+10
None or occasional	0

Score interpretation: ≥40: very likely pulmonary tuberculosis; 30-35: possibly pulmonary tuberculosis; ≤25: unlikely pulmonary tuberculosis. *BCG = Bacille Calmette-Guérin. Adapted from [5].

Worldwide, the most common symptoms of pediatric tuberculosis disease are a chronic cough for more than 21 days, a fever > 38 degrees C for 14 days (after common causes, such as malaria and pneumonia have been excluded), and weight loss or failure to thrive [6]. Active tuberculosis disease is most common under 5 years-old [7]. In young children, weight loss may be the only sign of disease. Adolescents, however, can exhibit typical B-cell symptoms, such as night sweats, fever, and lymphadenopathy. Additionally, hemoptysis and fatigue are more commonly experienced in adolescents than in younger children.

The diagnosis of perinatal tuberculosis is difficult because symptoms are also non-specific. These infants typically present 2-4 weeks of age with fever, respiratory distress, lethargy and tend to be commenced on broad spectrum antibiotics for presumed sepsis.

There are no pathognomonic signs on the physical examination that can confirm a diagnosis of tuberculosis. Some uncommon, but highly suggestive signs of pediatric tuberculosis include Gibbous deformity of the spine (or Pott's disease), non-painful lymphadenopathy, pleural or pericardial effusion, enlarged joints, and distended abdomen with ascites. A pneumonia or meningitis unresponsive to antibiotic treatment should also raise the suspicion of tuberculosis in endemic regions. Extrapulmonary tuberculosis disease is more common in children than adults, occurring in approximately 25% of infants and children less than 5 years-old [8]. The diagnosis of childhood tuberculosis is often based on the triad of (i) close contact with an infectious index case, (ii) a positive TST result, and (iii) observation of suggestive signs on a chest X-ray.

Diagnostic problems are more pronounced in HIV-infected children, and the performance of current diagnostic algorithms is poor in this group. Factors contributing to these additional diagnostic failure are varied: The lower sensitivity of TST in HIV-infected than in HIV-uninfected children, the chronic pulmonary symptoms that may be related to other HIV-related conditions (gastroesophageal reflux and bronchiecstasis) and a general reduction in the specificity of symptom-based diagnostic approaches. Furthermore, interpretation of chest X-ray is complicated by HIV-related co-morbidities, such as bacterial pneumonia, lymphocytic intersticial pneumonitis, bronchiectasis, pulmonary Kaposi sarcoma, and the atypical presentation of tuberculosis in immunecompromised children [9; 10].

Cerebrospinal fluid (CSF) findings are comparable in HIV-infected and HIV-uninfected patients with tuberculous meningitis. CSF white blood cell counts usually range from 100 to 500/mm^3, although some patients (15%) have > 500 white blood cells/mm^3. Lymphocyte predominance is typical, but 15-20% of patients have initial neutrophil predominance [11; 12]. CSF glucose values are usually depressed (<40 mg/dl in 80% of patients). CSF protein is almost always raised (75% of patients have values > 100 mg/dl), while opening pressures are elevated. In the absence of a definitive microbiological diagnosis, computed tomography (CT) can provide diagnostic certainty in most HIV-uninfected children. However, HIV-infected children are less likely to display the classic signs associated with tuberculous meningitis on head CT: Obstructive hydrocephalus (72% vs. 98%), basilar enhancement (38% vs. 71%), and parenchymal granulomas (0% vs. 15%) [13].

5.2. RADIOLOGICAL DIAGNOSIS

The diagnosis of tuberculosis in endemic areas depends predominantly on the subjective interpretation of the chest X-ray. Despite the limitations, radiological examinations remain the most practical and helpful test in everyday clinical practice. Chest X-ray changes are frequently nonspecific for tuberculosis. However, certain patterns, such as miliary disease, hilar adenopathy with airway compression and cavitary disease are associated with tuberculosis pulmonary disease [14]. A calcified lesion found in the pulmonary parenchyma indicates an old granuloma (Fig. **1**).

CT of the chest is more reliable when detecting adenopathy and pulmonary disease, but implies in much higher radiation exposure, being more expensive and also requires specialized expertise [14]. Chest X-rays of children with tuberculous meningitis are frequently abnormal, although a normal image cannot be used to exclude the disease. The most common radiographic findings are hilar adenopathy (60%), miliary pattern (20%), pleural effusion (15%), and cavitation (9%) [11; 13]. In plain X-rays, hilar lymphadenopathy is best seen on posteroanterior radiography as a lobulated density and can also be viewed in lateral films posterior to the bronchus intermedius. Miliary tuberculosis has the only distinct radiologically diagnostic feature of disease and is characterized by fine bilateral reticular shadowing, sometimes called a snowstorm appearance [15]. Since the signals are transient and not indicative of disease, it is imperative to evaluate the presence of other clinical signs and symptoms, and not to rely on the diagnosis of tuberculosis solely on the radiograph findings.

A more comprehensive description of this image method can be found in chapter 6.

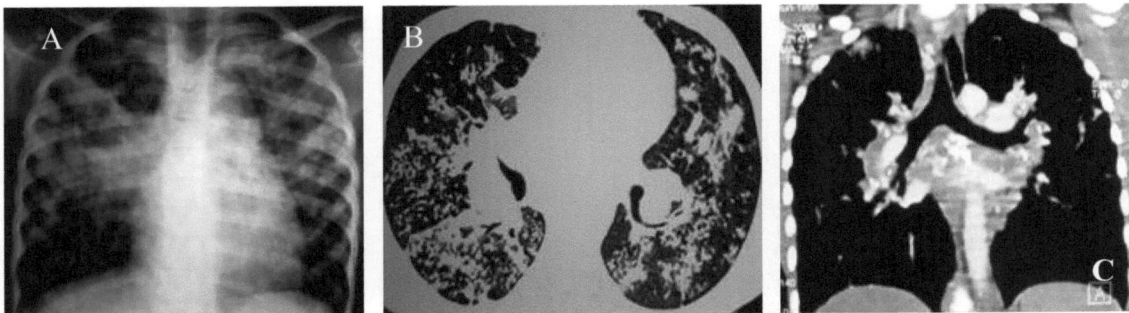

Fig. (1). (A) X-ray image of bilateral areas of consolidation and very bad-defined contours associated to right heart border with contour shadowed in a 10-years old patient first suspected of have Staph infection-associated pneumonia. Acid-fast bacilli yield positive result at sputum smear diagnosis. Household contact of an aunt with active pulmonary tuberculosis under treatment. (B) Computer tomography scan image showing foci of parenchimal consolidation in both lungs associated to signs of broncogenic dissemination characterized as air space nodules and peribronchial tree-in-bud pattern thickening. (C) Multiplanar computer tomography scan image in a coronal plane showing mediastinal enlargement with lymph nodes partially calcified.

5.3. BACTERIOLOGICAL DIAGNOSIS

As mentioned the gold standard, for the diagnosis of tuberculosis, is a positive culture of *M. tuberculosis* from biological specimens, such as sputum. In terms of bacteriological analysis, detection of acid-fast bacilli (AFB) in stained smears examined microscopically provides initial evidence of the presence of mycobacteria in a clinical specimen [16]. As standard culture with solid media requires up to 4-6 weeks, this method is not useful for diagnosis in a clinical setting. More rapid, liquid-based culture systems are becoming available, although due to costs and the need for specialized equipment and training they are not widely available in tuberculosis diagnostic clinics, especially in developing countries. In clinical practice, therefore, diagnosis relies more on direct microscopy of sputum to identify eventual cases of tuberculosis. Sputum smear-microscopy is relatively insensitive, because the presence of 10,000-100,000 organisms per ml is required for a positive result. Since children under 12 years-old do not often yield sputum and tend to swallow it, gastric aspiration is often used to obtain suspicious specimens. Suitable specimens from children are difficult to obtain, however, since a high proportion of childhood tuberculosis is extrapulmonary, it can require invasive procedures: Microbiological specimens, such as gastric aspirates, ascitic fluid, lymph node biopsy, endotracheal aspirate, bone marrow and cerebro-spinal fluid should be obtained, and stained and cultured for AFB. A typical positive AFB staining from sputum smear sample can be detected from an infected child (Fig. **2**).

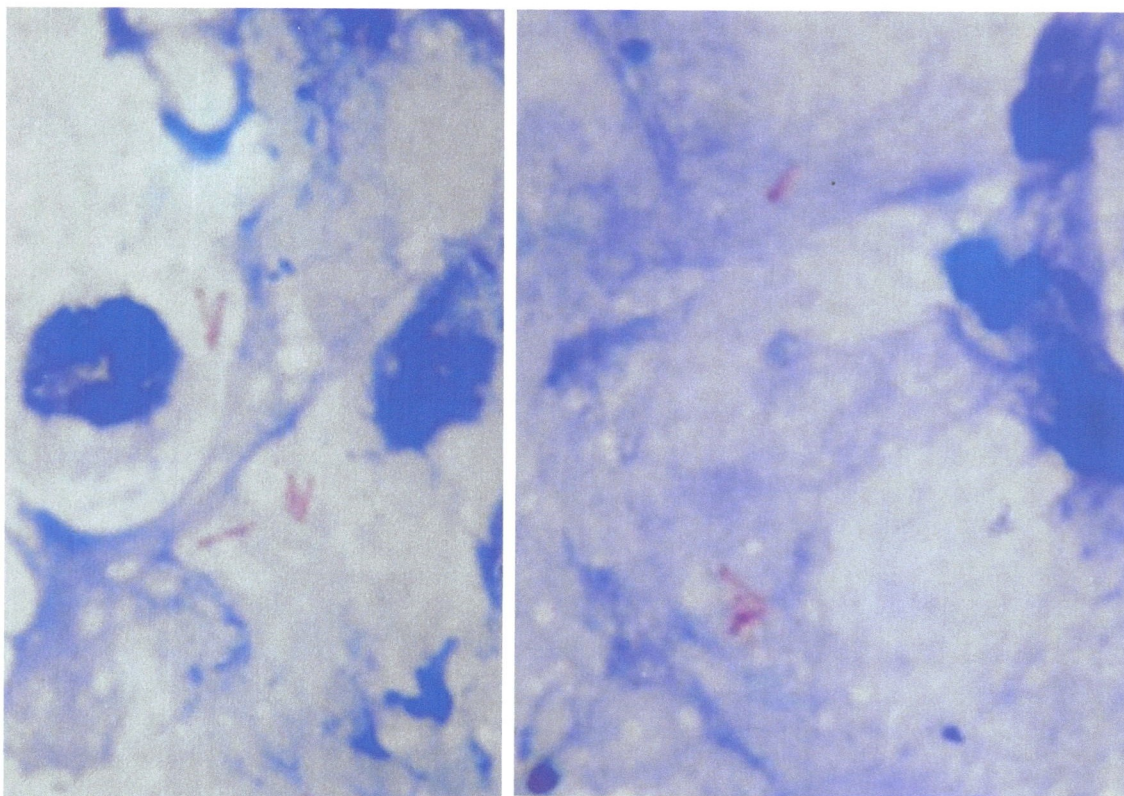

Fig. (2). The Ziehl-Neelsen staining technique showing two positive sputum smears in typical detections of acid-fast bacilli in children from bronchoalveolar lavage (x1,000).

AFB observed on smears may represent either *M. tuberculosis* or non-tuberculous mycobacteria (NTM). Because of the infectious potential of *M. tuberculosis*, acid-fast stains should be performed within 24 hours of receipt in the laboratory, and results should be reported to the physician immediately [17]. Specimens that are normally expected to be sterile, such as blood and urine, may be inoculated directly to conventional culture media. Conversely, specimens that may be contaminated with normal flora microorganisms require digestion and decontamination before inoculation to culture media to prevent overgrowth of these more rapidly replicating microbes. The use of a mucolytic agent (*e.g.* N-acetyl-l-cysteine) and a decontaminant (*e.g.* sodium hydroxide) is standard practice for respiratory and gastric specimens, but is not required for sterile site specimens, such as pleural fluid (Table **2**).

Table 2. Methods for Sample Decontamination.

Method	Use	Advantage	Disadvantage
Sodium hydroxide	- Laboratories using concentration by centrifugation.	- Digestion/ decontamination at the same time when used at a final concentration of 2%. - Low cost.	- Precise timing needed to avoid killing mycobacteria - may kill some mycobacteria even at 2% concentration.
N-acetyl-cysteine-sodium chloride-sodium hydroxide	- Most used in developed countries. - Used in combination with centrifugation.	- Good mucolytic action. - Use of NaCl as mucolytic reduces NaOH concentration and its potential deleterious action on mycobacteria.	- Short shelf-life of prepared reagents (24 h). - Higher cost.
Ogawa-Kudoh	- Ideal method for low resource settings	- Centrifugation or concentration is not necessary. - Low cost. - Can be used in the field.	- May have higher contamination rates.
Cetyl pyridinium - sodium chloride	- For preservation and digestion/ decontamination while in transport to the laboratory.	- Avoids overgrowth of contaminants for up to eight days.	- Egg-based media require since compound remains active in agar and may be deleterious to mycobacteria.

Adapted from [18].

General blood and other specimens prone to coagulate, including bone marrow, syno*via*l, pleural, pericardial and peritoneal fluids, should be collected in tubes containing sulfated polysaccharides or heparin. Sulfated polysaccharides are the preferred anticoagulants as they enhance the growth of mycobacteria [18]. Heparinized specimens are also satisfactory, but specimens collected in ethylenediaminetetraacetic acid (EDTA) are unacceptable, as even trace amounts of this chemical inhibit mycobacterial growth. Guidelines for collection of various types of specimens were adapted from Lighter and Rigaud (2009) and reproduced here (Table **3**).

Table 3. Specimens for Examination and Diagnostic Studies.

	Specimen	Procedure
1.	*Aspirates, fluids*	Sterile syringe, container, or direct inoculation to culture media.
2.	*Bone, bone marrow*	Direct inoculation to broth culture media designed for mycobacterial blood cultures or isolator tube.
3.	*Bronchial washings*	Sterile container.
4.	*Gastric washings*	Obtain when patient awakes; about 50 ml gastric aspirate in sterile container with 100 mg of sodium carbonate.
5.	*Sputum*	Exudates from lungs by a productive cough (not saliva), sterile container.
6.	*Stool*	Clear container.
7.	*Tissues, biopsy specimens*	Sterile container.
8.	*Urine*	First morning void, do not pool.

Source: [15].

Specimens should be transported rapidly to the laboratory to avoid overgrowth of other microorganisms. The cetylpyridinum chloride (CPC) method is widely used for the transport of sputum specimens [19], but the detection of AFB with Ziehl-Neelsen staining can be significantly reduced in specimens preserved by this method [20; 21]. In addition, specimens treated with CPC should be preferentially inoculated in egg-based media, because the agar-based media Middlebrook 7H9 and 7H10 have an insufficient neutralizing activity for this quaternary ammonium compound. Sodium carbonate was found to be a better preservative of sputum specimens for AFB smear microscopy, as well as for culture [22].

Gastric aspirates in neonates have a higher microbiological yield than in older infants (70%) and are well tolerated [23]. This procedure, as highlighted by Zar and colleagues (2005), is limited by a requirement for overnight fast, repeated specimens, attendance at the clinic and is uncomfortable for both the child and the health care worker. Collection of gastric content is best performed after a child has fasted for, at least, 8 hours and is still in bed. Aspiration is performed *via* silastic nasogastric tube, which is inserted before the child has taken anything by mouth. If unsuccessful, sterile distilled water can be instilled and aspirated. If gastric aspiration is performed under these conditions, *M. tuberculosis* can be recovered in up 50% of children with tuberculosis [25].

The yield from culture of 2-3 gastric aspirate samples obtained during fasting is ~30%-40% [24; 26; 27], although higher yields have been reported in cultures performed in children with advanced tuberculosis disease [28]. Alternative methods for sample collection include nasopharyngeal aspiration (which provides 30% yield vs. 38% yield noted with gastric aspiration), the string test and the sputum induction by mist hypertonic saline that has been reported to induce a higher yield of *M. tuberculosis* than gastric washings [24].

The string test is a novel approach that has been recently evaluated for its ability to retrieve *M. tuberculosis* from sputum-smear negative adults co-infected with HIV. A gelatin capsule that adheres to gastric contents over a couple of hours is swallowed, and then pulled back up for investigation. In Peru, the use of string test followed by sputum induction detected more cases of tuberculosis on culture of the specimens than did sputum induction alone [29]. It is well tolerated in children as young as 4 years-old, but further assessment of the bacteriologic yield and clinical utility in children remains to be seen.

Formal tissue biopsy may be important to exclude alternative diagnosis, particularly in children with mediastinal or intrathoracic nodal masses, when less invasive tests have not been successful. If tissue specimens are obtained, the examination by histological techniques as well as smear and culture is recommended [30]. Pleural tissue specimens were diagnostic by culture or histology in almost 80% of patients in whom biopsy was performed.

5.3.1. Microscopy

AFB microscopy has been shown to have sensitivity below 20% on gastric aspirate or sputum specimens from children [31; 32]. A negative microscopy result cannot exclude tuberculosis. Positive microscopy may be nonspecific due to the presence of NTM in patients with underlying structural lung disease, such as cystic fibrosis or bronchiectasis.

Traditional acid-fast staining techniques include the Ziehl-Neelsen and Kinyoun methods (Box 1). Fluorescent microscopy using Auramine O with or without Rhodamine B allows the scanning of slides at lower magnification and increase the sensitivity of the microscopy. While the reading of fuchsin-stained smears requires 1,000-fold magnification, fluorochrome-stained smears are examined at 250- or 450-fold. The lower magnification used in this staining methods allows the microscopist to observe a much larger area of the smear during the same period of time and thus, fewer fields must be read, reducing the laboratorist fatigue.

The increased sensitivity of fluorescence-stained AFB, over classical light microscopy for detection of pulmonary tuberculosis, has recently been confirmed in a systematic review of 45 studies. They compared the two methods in which fluorescence microscopy yielded an average increase in sensitivity of 10%, without loss of specificity [33]. However, the equipment costs for fluorescence microscopy are prohibitive, so use has been limited to regions that can afford it [15]. In addition, the fluorescence fades with time. For this reason, the slides must be read within 24 hours. A complete description of this approach can be found in chapter 7.

AFB staining of CSF is frequently negative. The sensitivity may be increased by collecting large volumes of fluid (5-10 ml) with subsequent centrifugation, or by repeated sampling; CSF cultures are usually positive for *M. tuberculosis* in approximately one-third of cases, and sputum or gastric aspirate cultures are positive in 50% of children [Reviewed by 34].

Box 1. Principle of Staining Acid-Fast Bacilli.

Mycobacterial cell walls contain a waxy substance composed of mycolic acids. These are β-hydroxy carboxylic acids with chain lengths of up to 90 carbon atoms. The property of acid fastness is related to the carbon chain length of the mycolic acid found in any particular species. Basic fuchsin binds to negatively charged groups in bacteria. The mycolic acid (and other cell wall lipids) presents a barrier to dye entry as well as elusion (washing out with solvent) and this is partly overcome by adding a lipophilic agent to a concentrated aqueous solution of basic fuchsin and partly by heating.

When viewed under a microscope, the stained slide will show acid-fast organisms as red and nonacid-fast organisms as blue. The traditional acid-fast staining techniques are: Ziehl-Neelsen and Kinyoun. The procedure for both techniques is similar, but unlike Ziehl-Neelsen stain, the Kinyoun method does not involve heating the slides being stained.

5.3.2. Culture

Culture is more sensitive than microscopy, and can detect as few as 10 to 100 bacteria/ml of material [35], but it is positive in less than 50% of children with active tuberculosis disease. In the U.S.A., 90% of tuberculosis cases in adults were bacteriologically confirmed from 1985 to 1988, compared to only 28% in children [36]. Culture of the organism allows drug susceptibility testing and is therefore most critical where drug resistance is of concern for epidemiological reasons [7]. In general, the sensitivity of culture-based mycobacteria detection is 80-85%, and the specificity is approximately 98% [37; 38].

Mycobacterial culture may be performed using solid media, such as the egg-based Lowenstein-Jensen (LJ) slopes or the Middlebrook series of agars, or using liquid broths [30] (Table **3**). The Ogawa medium is another egg-based medium, which is comparable on its composition to LJ. It is more economic because it replaces asparagines with sodium glutamate, an amino acid more readily available and much cheaper.

Liquid culture media has been proven to be significantly more sensitive than egg-based solid media for the isolation of mycobacteria from clinical specimens [39].

LJ medium has been used for culture of *M. tuberculosis* in resource-challenge countries. To establish resistant *M. tuberculosis* isolates, Middlebrook 7H11 is better than LJ. Once a colony appears, physiologic tests are performed to identify mycobacterial species. Isolation of a NTM of potential clinical significance is not *ipso facto* evidence that the patient's disease manifestation is caused by the NTM. Each mycobacterial isolate, like each patient, must be evaluated individually [40]. Such approaches include pigment inspection, microscopy examination for cording, and colony morphology. Also, this can be accomplished by biochemical tests to distinguish mycobacterial species, but such tests are time-consuming and laborious. A more reliable method for identifying mycobacteria is the use of chromatography for the analysis of fatty acids with typical moieties extracted from the mycobacterial cell wall [15]. High Performance Liquid Chromatography (HPLC) can replace an entire battery of biochemical tests. HPLC differentiates mycobacteria according to their species-specific synthesis of mycolic acids, β-hydroxy-α-fatty acids that are components of the cell wall [41]. The limitation of this technique is that HPLC cannot distinguish *M. tuberculosis* from *M. bovis*, although it can differentiate *M. bovis* Bacille Calmette-Guérin (BCG) and *M. tuberculosis* complex.

Liquid media support growth of the *M. tuberculosis* complex better than solid media (Table **4**). The first broth-based mycobacterial detection system was BACTEC 460, which uses a modified Middlebrook broth and a radiometric detection scheme. A non-radiometric liquid culture system has been developed to minimize the handling and disposal of radioactive waste [42]. More recently, liquid culture medium (MGIT), in which an indicator dye changes colour with growth, provided culture results more quickly, within 2-4 weeks. The MGIT processes all types of clinical specimens other than blood and urine; however, previous results demonstrated high sensitivity when using concentrated urine specimens [43].

Table 4. Comparison Between Liquid and Solid Media in Diagnosis of Child Tuberculosis.

Medium	Liquid Media	Solid Media
Types of Media	BACTEC 460 *Mycobacterial Growth Indicator Tube (MGIT)*	*egg-based: e.g. Lowenstein-Jensen (LJ contains malachite green that suppresses growth of contaminating bacteria and fungi, and is used for both detection and susceptibility testing).* *agar-based: e.g. Middlebrook 7H10 and 7H11.*
Time for detection	*2 and 4 weeks for isolation and susceptibility test, respectively.*	*3 and 4 weeks.*
Advantages	*Support growth of the M. tuberculosis complex better than solid media with an increased recovery of positive cultures, even in cases in which a child was started on anti-tuberculosis medication before obtaining cultures.* *It demands shorter time to detection of positive cultures than in solid media. The average time to recovery for smear-positive specimens is only 8 days compared to 18 days for solid conventional media.*	*Allows the determination of characteristic features of colonial morphology, growth rate, and pigment production.*
Disadvantages	*Excessive cost*	*Sub-optimal sensitivity, slow turn around times.*

5.4. IMMUNOLOGICAL DIAGNOSIS

The Tuberculin Skin Test (TST) is widely used to support clinical and radiological findings during the evaluation of children with suspected tuberculosis. In 1934, the American scientist Dr. Florence Siebert developed a method of purifying the tuberculin, and made a simple protein precipitate, a solution of crude antigens produced by the metabolic activity of *M. tuberculosis*. The TST is based on the detection of a cutaneous delayed-type hypersensitivity response to purified protein derivative (PPD), a poorly defined mixture of antigens presented in *M. tuberculosis*, *M. bovis* BCG and several NTM. Today, the definitive TST uses five tuberculin units of PPD injected intradermally in the forearm, the so-called Mantoux technique. A wheal of fluid measuring 6 to 10 mm in diameter is raised immediately when the tuberculin is injected properly. A delayed-type hypersensitivity reaction to the TST peaks in infected individuals at 48 to 72 hours after injection. The diameter of induration, not erythema, is measured and recorded in millimeters. A positive TST result may help in decision to start treatment while bacteriological confirmation is awaited or when it is lacking. This assay is relatively cheap and does not require a laboratory, but presents numerous limitations. A typical positive TST can be easily detected and read in an infected child forearm (Fig. **3**).

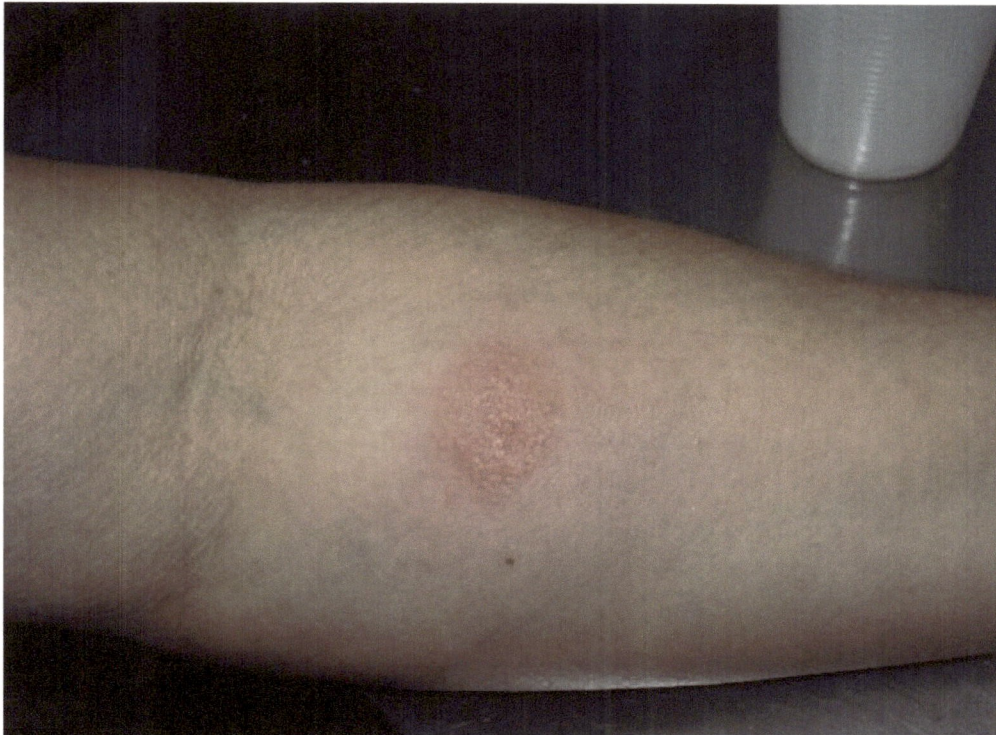

Fig. (3). A positive tuberculin skin test in an infected child forearm showing an important area with a phlyctenular aspect.

The TST has several complications in realization, and also in lecture. A negative TST does not necessarily exclude infection with *M. tuberculosis*. There are many factors that can cause a decreased response to TST, including concurrent illnesses or infections, along with active tuberculosis. Up to 25% of people with active tuberculosis are nonreactive to the five tuberculin units [44]. The sensitivity is default in several circumstances (malnutrition, viruses or bacterial infections, immunological deficiencies, children above 2 years-old, and others). In addition, the false-negative rate is increased by the failure to administer the PPD intradermally, and also the complexity encountered in reading the indurated reaction of the test (Table **5**).

Table 5. Causes of False-Positive or False-Negative Tuberculin Skin Tests (TST) in Children.

False-negative TST	False-positive TST
Improper placing/interpretation	
HIV infection	
Malnutrition or low-protein states	
Severe tuberculosis	
Improper storage of tuberculin	Improper interpretation
Viral infections	BCG vaccination
Bacterial infections	Non-tuberculous mycobacteria
Live viral vaccines (within 6 weeks)	
Immunedeficiencies	
Neonates	

The TST positivity is based on the size of induration and epidemiologic risk factors. The USA Centers for Disease Control and Prevention (CDC) and the American Academy of Physician recommend specific interpretations of skin reactions (Table **6**). The specificity of TST is difficult where BCG vaccination is generalized. About 50% of infants vaccinated with BCG will have a positive TST, yet 80 to 90% lose such reactivity within 2 to 3 years. In fact, if BCG is given in the newborn period, less than 5% of children will exhibit a cross-reaction by 10 years-old [45; 46]. PPD contains over 200 antigens shared with the BCG vaccine and most NTM [47]. A meta-analysis found that the TST false-positive rate in children from NTM is about 2% [46]. In addition, sensitivity of TST in young children is unknown, and because of this uncertainty, along with the confounding effect of BCG in vaccinated children, guidelines for the interpretation of TST results in child tuberculosis contacts vary widely. TST may be negative in up to 40% of HIV-negative children presenting with extrapulmonary tuberculosis [13], compounding the difficulties during diagnosis of young children.

Table 6. Definitions of Positive Tuberculin Skin Tests Results in Infants, Children and Adolescents.

Induration ≥ 5 mm

Children in close contact with known or suspected contagious people with tuberculosis disease.

Children suspected to have tuberculosis disease:

- *Findings on chest radiograph consistent with active or previously tuberculosis disease*
- *Clinical evidence of tuberculosis disease*

Children receiving immunesuppressive therapy or with immunesuppressive conditions, including HIV infection.

Induration ≥ 10 mm

Children at increased risk of disseminated tuberculosis disease:

- *Children younger than 4 years-old*
- *Children with other medical conditions, including Hodgkin disease, lymphoma, diabetes mellitus, chronic renal failure, or malnutrition*

Children with increased exposure to tuberculosis disease:

- *Children born in high-prevalence regions of the world*
- *Children frequently exposed to adults who are HIV infected, homeless, users of illicit drugs, residents or nursing homes, incarcerated or institutionalized, or migrant farm workers*
- *Children who travel to high-prevalence regions of the world.*

Induration ≥ 15 mm

Children 4 years-old or older without any risk factors.

Source: [15].

Immune-based tests would seem to offer the potential to improve case detection as currently performed, as some of the tests formats are suitable for resource-limited settings. The major advantages of immune-based tests are their speed and simplicity compared to microscopy [48-51]. The development of immune-based tests for the detection of antibodies, antigens, and immune complexes has been attempted for decades.

The most common of these tests rely on detection of the humoral immune response to *M. tuberculosis,* as opposed to the T cell-based immune response, or direct detection of antigens in specimens other than serum. Several serological tests for tuberculosis have been developed recently using a variety of *M. tuberculosis* antigens to detect certain antibodies in the circulation, including complement fixation tests, hemagglutination tests, radioimmunoassay and ELISAs [15]. These tests differ in a number of their features, including antigen composition, antigen source, chemical composition, extend and manner of purification of the antigen and class of immunoglobulin detected (IgG, IgM or IgA) [33]. No serological test has been widely implemented in clinical care. Children tend to have lower antibody titers than adults which represent a particular problem for the use of serological tests in the pediatric population [52].

Steingart and colleagues (2007) reviewed the accuracy of available antibody detection tests for the diagnosis of pulmonary tuberculosis. They concluded that there are insufficient data to determine the accuracy of most commercial tests, in smear microscopy-negative patients, as well as their performance in children (usually smear-negative) and persons with HIV infection. These tests cannot distinguish latent from active tuberculosis disease, and several factors may affect their reliability, such as BCG vaccination, and HIV- and NTM-infections [14].

Only a few published studies report on antibody detection in primary infection, a condition that predominantly occurs in children [15]. Some authors have found a sensitivity of 84% and 73% for the 30 and 16 kDa antigens, respectively [53]. In addition, a study in India showed the 38 kDa antigen to be positive in 37% of children with pulmonary tuberculosis, 86% with tuberculous lymphadenitis, and 27% of controls (possibly with latent infection) [54].

The currently available serological assays are highly variable in their sensitivity and specificity. Furthermore, serological assays are limited as antibody responses are variable, while the antibody detection test can be developed into a number of formats: Common designs include the ELISA and the immunochromatographic test format.

5.5. BIOCHEMICAL DIAGNOSIS

M. tuberculosis also can be identified by its rough, non-pigmented, corded colonies on oleic acid-albumin agars; a positive niacin accumulation test; generally weak catalase activity that is lost completely by heating to 68 degrees C; and a positive nitrate reduction test.

5.5.1. Niacin Accumulation Test

M. tuberculosis excretes niacin due a blockade in their scavenging pathway. The excreted niacin accumulates in the culture medium and is evidenced in the presence of cyanogens halide with a primary amine. Niacin-negative *M. tuberculosis* strains are extremely rare.

5.5.2. Nitrate Reduction Test

This test is particularly useful for differentiating *M. tuberculosis*, which gives a positive reaction, from *M. bovis*, which is negative [55; 56].

5.5.3. Catalase Test

M. tuberculosis gives negative results, as do other species in the *M. tuberculosis* complex. Catalase is an intracellular enzyme that transforms hydrogen peroxide to oxygen and water.

5.5.4. Pyrazinamidase Test

Pyrazinamidase is an enzyme that hydrolyzes pyrazinamide to ammonia and pyrazinoic acid. This test is useful to differentiate *M. tuberculosis* (positive) from the other species of the *M. tuberculosis* complex, with exception of *M. canetti*.

5.5.5. Growth in the Presence of Thiophen-2-Carboxylic acid Hydrazide

This test is useful to distinguish *M. tuberculosis*, which grows in the presence of this compound, from other members of the *M. tuberculosis* complex. Most NTM are also positive to this test.

5.5.6. Adenosine Deaminase Activity

Adenosine deaminase (ADA) is an enzyme involved in the metabolism of purines. Many studies have reported the utility of ADA determinations in body fluids (spinal, pleural, ascetic, pericardial) for the diagnosis of tuberculous meningitis [57; 58], tuberculous pleurisy [59-61], peritoneal tuberculosis [62; 63] and pericardial tuberculosis [64-66]. AFB may be difficult to isolate from these specimens because they are often diluted in large fluid volumes. ADA determination is simple and cheap, and also has a high positive predictive value, especially in high endemic countries. The specificity is very high in fluids with a lymphocyte-to-neutrophil ratio higher than 0.75 [67, 68].

5.6. MOLECULAR DIAGNOSIS

Newer modalities, such as polymerase chain reaction (PCR) and restriction fragment length polymorphisms (RFLP), can be useful for diagnosis and identification of the index case. Studies have reported poor sensitivity of PCR in paucibacillary disease and also in extrapulmonary tuberculosis, but yield good specificity. In smear-negative disease, sensitivity is around 50-60% but specificity approaches 99%. In general, PCR is less sensitive than culture, and is limited by cost and need for laboratory expertise and infrastructure [14]. However, because biochemical methods generally lack rapidity and ease of use, the nucleic acid amplification test (NAAT) can be substituted. NAATs use molecular probes that can hybridize specifically with *M. tuberculosis* complex, *M. avium* complex, *M. kansasii*, or *M. gordonae* [69]. These assays exhibit sensitivities and specificities approaching 100% when at least 100,000 organisms are present.

A complete description of this molecular method can be found in chapter 7.

REFERENCES

[1] World Health Organization. Global Tuberculosis Control: Surveillance, Planning, Financing. 2002. Report No. 2002.

[2] Brazilian Ministry of Health. Tuberculose: guia de vigilância epidemiológica. Brasília, Brazil; 2002. Report.

[3] Hesseling AC, Schaaf HS, Gie RP, Starke JR, Beyers N. A critical review of diagnostic approaches in the diagnosis of childhood tuberculosis. Int J Tuberc Lung Dis 2002; 6: 1038-45.

[4] World Health Organization. Guidance for National Tuberculosis Programs on the Management of Tuberculosis in Children. 2006. Report No. 2006.

[5] Maciel EL, Dietze R, Silva RE, Hadad DJ, Struchiner CJ. Evaluation of a scoring system recommended by the Brazilian Ministry of Health for the diagnosis of childhood tuberculosis. Cad Saude Publica 2008; 24: 402-8.

[6] World Health Organization. Communicable diseases: tuberculosis fact sheet. Tuberculosis and children. 2008. Report No. 2008.

[7] Snider DEJ, Rieder HL, Combs D, Bloch AB, Hayden CH, Smith MH. Tuberculosis in children. Pediatr Infect Dis J 1988; 7: 271-8.

[8] Jacobs RF, Starke JR. Tuberculosis in children. Med Clin North Am 1993; 77: 1335-51.

[9] Graham SM, Coulter JB, Gilks CF. Pulmonary disease in HIV-infected African children. Int J Tuberc Lung Dis 2001; 5: 12-23.

[10] Marais BJ, Graham SM, Cotton MF, Beyers N. Diagnostic and management challenges for childhood tuberculosis in the era of HIV. J Infect Dis 2007; 196: 76-85.

[11] Topley JM, Bamber S, Coovadia HM, Corr PD. Tuberculosis meningitis and co-infection with HIV. Ann Trop Paediatr 1998; 18: 261-6.

[12] Yaramis A, Gurkan F, Elevli M, *et al.* Central nervous system tuberculosis in children: a review of 214 cases. Pediatrics 1998; 102: 49.

[13] van der Weert EM, Hartgers NM, Schaaf HS, *et al.* Comparison of diagnostic criteria of tuberculosis meningitis in human immunodeficiency virus-infected and uninfected children. Pediatr Infect Dis J 2006; 25: 65-9.

[14] Zar HJ. Diagnosis of pulmonary tuberculosis in children: what's new? S. Afr. Med J 2007; 97: 983-5.

[15] Lighter J, Rigaud M. Diagnosing childhood tuberculosis: traditional and innovative modalities. Curr Probl Pediatr Adolesc Health Care 2009; 39: 61-88.

[16] American Thoracic Society, Centers for Disease Control and Prevention. Diagnostic standards and classification of tuberculosis in adults and children. Am J Respir Crit Care Med; 2000. Report No.: 161.

[17] Association of State and Territorial Public Health Laboratory Directors and the Centers for Disease Control and Prevention. *Mycobacterium tuberculosis*: assessing your laboratory. Washington, D.C.: U.S. Government Printing Office; 1995. Report.

[18] Waard JH, Robledo J. Conventional Diagnostic Methods. Tuberculosis Book. 2007. pp. 401-24.

[19] Smithwick RW, Stratigos CB, David HL. Use of cetylpyridinium chloride and sodium chloride for the decontamination of sputum specimens that are transported to the laboratory for the isolation of *Mycobacterium tuberculosis*. J Clin Microbiol 1975; 1: 411-3.

[20] Selvakumar N, Sudhamathi S, Duraipandian M, Frieden TR, Narayanan PR. Reduced detection by Ziehl-Neelsen method of acid-fast bacilli in sputum samples preserved in cetylpyridinum chloride solution. Int J Tuberc Lung Dis 2004; 8: 248-52.

[21]   Selvakumar N, Gomathi Sekar M, Kumar V, Bhaskar Rao DV, Rahman F, Narayanan PR. Sensitivity of Ziehl-Neelsen method for centrifuged deposit smears of sputum samples transported in cetyl-pyridinium chloride. Indian J Med Res 2006; 124: 439-42.

[22]   Bobadilla-del-Valle M, Ponce-de-Leon A, Kato-Maeda M, *et al.* Comparison of sodium carbonate, cetil-pyridinium chloride, and sodium borate for preservation of sputa for culture of *Mycobacterium tuberculosis.* J Clin Microbiol 2003; 41: 4487-8.

[23]   Vallejo JG, Ong LT, Starke JR. Clinical features, diagnosis, and treatment of tuberculosis in infants. Pediatrics 1994; 94: 1-7.

[24]   Zar HJ, Hanslo D, Apolles P, Swingler G, Hussey G. Induced sputum versus gastric lavage for microbiological confirmation of pulmonary tuberculosis in infants and young children: a prospective study. Lancet 2005; 365: 130-4.

[25]   Pomputius WF, III, Rost J, Dennehy PH, Carter EJ. Standardization of gastric aspirate technique improves yield in the diagnosis of tuberculosis in children. Pediatr Infect Dis J 1997; 16(2): 222-6.

[26]   Eamranond P, Jaramillo E. Tuberculosis in children: reassessing the need for improved diagnosis in global control strategies. Int J Tuberc Lung Dis 2001; 5: 594-603.

[27]   Starke JR. Pediatric tuberculosis: time for a new approach. Tuberculosis 2003; 83: 208-12.

[28]   Marais BJ, Brittle W, Painczyk K, *et al.* Use of light-emitting diode fluorescence microscopy to detect acid-fast bacilli in sputum. Clin Infect Dis 2008; 47: 203-7.

[29]   Vargas D, Garcia L, Gilman RH, *et al.* Diagnosis of sputum-scarce HIV-associated pulmonary tuberculosis in Lima, Peru. Lancet 2005; 365: 150-2.

[30]   Andresen D. Microbiological diagnostic procedures in respiratory infections: mycobacterial infections. Paediatr Respir Rev 2007; 8: 221-30.

[31]   Starke JR, Taylor-Watts KT. Tuberculosis in the pediatric population of Houston, Texas. Pediatrics 1989; 84: 28-35.

[32]   Starke JR. Childhood tuberculosis: A diagnostic dilemma (Editorial). Chest 1993; 104: 329-30.

[33]   Steingart KR, Laal S, Hopewell PC, *et al.* Commercial serological antibody detection tests for the diagnosis of pulmonary tuberculosis: a systematic review. PLoS Med 2007; 4: 202.

[34]   Rowe JS, Shah SS, Marais BJ, Steenhoff AP. Diagnosis and management of tuberculous meningitis in HIV-infected pediatric patients. Pediatr Infect Dis J 2009; 28: 147-8.

[35]   Yeager HJ, Lacy J, Smith LR, LeMaistre CA. Quantitative studies of mycobacterial populations in sputum and saliva. Am Rev Respir Dis 1967; 95: 998-1004.

[36]   Braun M. Pediatric tuberculosis, bacilli Calmette-Guerin immunization, and acquired immunodeficiency syndrome. Semin Infect Dis 1993; 4: 261-8.

[37]   Morgan MA, Horstmeier CD, DeYoung DR, Roberts GD. Comparison of a radiometric method (BACTEC) and conventional culture media for recovery of mycobacteria from smear-negative specimens. J Clin Microbiol 1983; 18: 384-8.

[38]   Ichiyama S, Shimokata K, Takeuchi J, the AMR group. Comparative study of a biophasic culture system (Roche MB check system) with a conventional egg medium for recovery of mycobacteria. Tuber Lung Dis 1993; 74: 338-41.

[39]   Hines N. Comparison of the recovery of *Mycobacterium bovis* isolates using the BACTEC MGIT 960 system, BACTEC 460 system, and Middlebrook 7H10 and 7H11 solid media. J Vet Diagn Invest 2006; 18: 243-50.

[40]   American Thoracic Society. Diagnosis and treatment of disease caused by non-tuberculous mycobacteria. Am J Respir Crit Care Med; 1997. Report No.: 156.

[41]   Butler WR, Kilburn JO. Identification of major slowly growing pathogenic mycobacteria and *Mycobacterium gordonae* by high performance liquid chromatography of their mycolic acids. J Clin Microbiol 1988; 26: 50-3.

[42]   Hanna BA. Laboratory diagnosis. In: Rom WN, Garay SM, editors. Tuberculosis. 2nd ed. Lippincott, Williams and Wilkins. Philadelphia 2004. pp. 164-76.

[43]   Chan PC, Chang LY, Wu YC, *et al.* Age-specific cut-offs for the tuberculin skin test to detect latent tuberculosis in BCG-vaccinated children. Int J Tuberc Lung Dis 2008; 12: 1401-6.

[44]   Nash DR, Douglass JE. Anergy in active pulmonary tuberculosis: A comparison between positive and negative reactors and an evaluation of 5 TU and 250 TU skin test doses. Chest 1980; 77: 32-7.

[45]   Menzies R, Vissandjee B, Amyot D. Factors associated with tuberculin reactivity among the foreign-born in Montreal. Am Rev Respir Dis 1992; 146: 752-6.

[46]   Farhat M, Greenaway C, Pai M, Menzies D. False-positive tuberculin skin tests: what is the absolute effect of BCG and non-tuberculous mycobacteria? Int J Tuberc Lung Dis 2006; 10: 1192-204.

[47] Huebner RE, Good RC, Tokars JI. Current practices in mycobacteriology: results of a survey of state public health laboratories. J Clin Microbiol 1993; 31(4): 771-5.

[48] Elliott A. Diagnosis and treatment of tuberculosis in children. Trop Doct 1993; 23: 142-3.

[49] Johnson JL, Vjecha MJ, Okwera A, *et al.* Management of tuberculosis. Int J Tuberc Lung Dis 1998; 2: 397-404.

[50] Shingadia D, Novelli V. Diagnosis and treatment of tuberculosis in children. Lancet Infect Dis 2003; 3: 624-32.

[51] Perkins MD, Roscigno G, Zumla A. Progress towards improved tuberculosis diagnostics for developing countries. Lancet 2006; 367: 942-3.

[52] Mahadevan S. Impact of human immunodeficiency virus type-1 infection on the initial bacteriologic and radiographic manifestations of pulmonary tuberculosis in Uganda. Indian J Pediatr 1997; 64: 97-103.

[53] Raja A, Ranganathan UD, Bethunaickan R, Dharmalingam V. Clinical utility of serodiagnosis of tuberculosis. Pediatr Infect Dis J 2001; 20: 1161-4.

[54] Swaminathan S, Umadevi P, Shantha S, Radhakrishnan A, Datta M. Serodiagnosis of tuberculosis in children using two ELISA kits. Indian J Pediatr 1999; 66: 837-42.

[55] Tsukamura M, Shimoide H, Kita N, Kawakami K, Kuze A. Relationship between prevalence rates of non-tuberculous lung mycobacteriosis and active lung tuberculosis. Geographic difference of the prevalence rate of non-tuberculous lung mycobacteriosis. Kekkaku 1984; 59(2): 105-13.

[56] Vincent V, Marchal G. *Mycobacterium tuberculosis* and its host. Rev Prat 2002; 52(19): 2111-4.

[57] Lopez-Cortes LF, Cruz-Ruiz M, Gomez-Mateos J, *et al.* Adenosine deaminase activity in the CSF of patients with aseptic meningitis: utility in the diagnosis of tuberculous meningitis or neurobrucellosis. Clin Infect Dis 1995; 20: 525-30.

[58] Kashyap RS, Kainthia RP, Mudaliar AV, Purohit HJ, Taori GM, Daginawala HF. Cerebrospinal fluid adenosine deaminase activity: a complimentary tool in the early diagnosis of tuberculous meningitis. Cerebrospinal Fluid Res 2006; 30: 3-5.

[59] Banales JL. Adenosine deaminase in the diagnosis of tuberculous pleural effusions: A report of 218 patients and review of the literature. Chest 1991; 99: 355-7.

[60] Perez-Rodriguez E, Jimenez Castro D. The use of adenosine deaminase activity and adenosine deaminase isoenzymes in the diagnosis of tuberculous pleuritis. Curr Opin Pulm Med 2000; 6: 259-66.

[61] Goto M, Noguchi Y, Koyama H, Hira K, Shimbo T, Fukui T. Diagnostic value of adenosine deaminase in tuberculous pleural effusion: a meta-analysis. Ann Clin Biochem 2003; 40: 374-81.

[62] Aston NO. Abdominal tuberculosis. World J Surg 1997; 21: 492-9.

[63] Gilroy D, Sherigar J. Concurrent small bowel lymphoma and mycobacterial infection: use of adenosine deaminase activity and polymerase chain reaction to facilitate rapid diagnosis and treatment. Eur J Gastroenterol Hepatol 2006; 18: 305-7.

[64] Reuter H, Burgess LJ, Carstens ME, Doubell AF. Characterization of the immunological features of tuberculous pericardial effusions in HIV positive and HIV negative patients in contrast with non-tuberculous effusions. Tuberculosis (Edinb) 2006; 86(2): 125-33.

[65] Reuter H, Burgess L, van Vuuren W, Doubell A. Diagnosing tuberculosis pericarditis. QJM 2006; 99: 827-39.

[66] Tuon FF, Litvoc MN, Lopes MI. Adenosine deaminase and tuberculous pericarditis: a systematic review with meta-analysis. Acta Trop 2006; 99: 67-74.

[67] Burgess LJ, Maritz FJ, Le R, I, Taljaard JJ. Combined use of pleural adenosine deaminase with lymphocyte/neutrophil ratio. Increased specificity for the diagnosis of tuberculous pleuritis. Chest 1996; 109(2): 414-9.

[68] Diacon AH, Van de Wal BW, Wyser C, *et al.* Diagnostic tools in tuberculous pleurisy: a direct comparative study. Eur Respir J 2003; 22: 589-91.

[69] Shinnick T, Good R. Diagnostic mycobacteriology laboratory practices. Clin Infect Dis 1995; 21: 291-9.

CHAPTER 6

Radiology in Pulmonary Tuberculosis

Almério S. Machado Jr.[1,*] and Paulo R.Z. Antas[2]

[1]*Escola Bahiana de Medicina e Saúde Pública, Av. Dom João VI, # 274, Brotas Nazaré; zip: 40.290-000, Salvador, Bahia, Brazil and* [2]*Laboratório de Imunologia Clínica, Fiocruz, Av. Brasil, # 4365; zip: 21045-900, Rio de Janeiro, Brazil*

Abstract: Pulmonary tuberculosis is a common worldwide infection, causing high mortality and morbidity, especially in developing countries. Despite advances in diagnosis of tuberculosis, chest imaging, combined with the clinical history, remain the basis in the diagnosis, staging and follow-up of pulmonary tuberculosis. Typical radiological patterns of pulmonary tuberculosis help clinicians in management of the disease. Upper zone shadows, frequently bilateral and often associated with cavitation, are typical, as are miliary lesions. However, these findings are uncommon in childhood thoracic tuberculosis. The diagnosis of childhood intrathoracic tuberculosis depends on a constellation of symptoms, signs, and tuberculin skin test and chest radiograph results. Paratracheal, mediastinal, and hilar lymphadenopathy are frequent in childhood tuberculosis. In HIV-infected patients the radiological appearances are less specific, just as symptoms and signs may not be typical and sputum is often negative on direct smear. However chest computed tomography (CT) is frequently necessary to establish the need of additional tests. CT is more sensitive than chest X-ray in the detection and characterization of both slight localized or disseminated parenchymal disease and mediastinal lymphadenopathy. Eventually, nuclear medicine can be necessary since it provides tools for diagnosis and monitoring tuberculosis mainly in children, HIV immunecompromised individuals, tuberculosis sequel and suspected reactivation.

Keywords: Childhood Intrathoracic Tuberculosis, Radiological Diagnosis, Cavitation, Chest Computer Tomography, Nuclear Medicine.

6.1. BACKGROUND

Wilhelm Conrad Röntgen's discovery of X-rays occurred in 1895, when he studied a cathode ray tube enclosed within an opaque cardboard container [1]. At that time, pulmonary tuberculosis was responsible for hundreds of thousands of deaths around the world. This innovation allowed introduction of screening rooms in medical procedures, including evaluation of thoracic diseases. In 1899, Bouchard was first to note tuberculous pleural effusion, and Walsman described lung cavities and miliary disease. At the end of the World War I, tuberculosis spread around the world with huge intensity. This way, adoption of disease control measures became required. These actions included the identification of patients through X-ray, which intensified the use of this image method in several countries [2-4]. Since then, chest X-rays have been used routinely in the initial diagnosis of pulmonary tuberculosis in adults and children.

6.2. TUBERCULOSIS PATHOGENESIS

Pulmonary tuberculosis is divided into primary and secondary infections. The primary form occurs in individuals who have not yet contacted the bacillus. It is more common in children. The secondary form develops from a new infection (exogenous) or re-infection, or from the reactivation of latent bacilli (endogenous) [5].

In the primary infection, inhaled *Mycobacterium tuberculosis* reaches deep portions of the lung and invades resident macrophages in pulmonary alveoli [3]. The initial events following infection have been extensively

Address correspondence to Almério S. Machado Jr.: Escola Bahiana de Medicina e Saúde Pública, Av. Dom João VI, # 274, Brotas Nazaré; zip: 40.290-000, Salvador, Bahia, Brazil; Tel: +55 71 2101-2900, Fax: +55 71 3356-1936, E-mail: almeriojr@yahoo.com.br

Paulo Renato Zuquim Antas, Dilvani Oliveira Santos, Roberta Olmo Pinheiro and Theolis Barbosa (Eds)

studied in the mouse model. Infected macrophages attract uninfected tissue macrophages, blood monocytes, lymphocytes and dendritic cells, a process that is dependent of sustained tumor necrosis factor (TNF)-signaling by the infected macrophages [6]. Stimulated by interaction with T lymphocytes, macrophages differentiate into epithelioid histiocytes [7]. This ensemble of lymphoid cells aggregate around the infected macrophages, forming a core of foamy macrophages and multinucleated giant cells, surrounded by lymphocytes and contained within a fibrous cuff of collagen and extracellular matrix components that "wall off" the structure, isolating it from the parenchymal tissue [6]. This constitutes the primary granuloma, where bacilli are believed to be contained from dissemination to other areas of the lung. However, some studies indicate that mycobacteria may escape the granuloma even in the absence of reactivation disease, and viable bacilli can be recovered from lung parenchyma of healthy individuals [8].

The set of primary granulomas receive the name of Ghon's focus. Primary tuberculosis complex is the solid set of Ghon's focus, lymphangitis and lymphadenitis. Depending on the number and virulence of bacilli as well as hypersensitivity and degree of resistance, host can evolve to cure or to disease [5].

The primary disease evolves from the pulmonary focus or from a pneumonic process. Lymph nodes involvement may create fistulae from an adjacent bronchus and determine bronchogenic tuberculosis. With the expansion of the destructive lesions, the bacilli reach blood vessels and spread to the lung and other organs [5].

The initial lesion, or a new parenchymal infection, can originate central necrosis and liquefaction and elimination of material from a bronchus. From the cavity structure, bacilli can spread to the lung through the bronchial tree (bronchogenic spread) and, as occurs in childhood, by hematogenous spread (miliary tuberculosis) [5]. The readers should refer to chapter 2 for a more detailed review on tuberculosis pathogenesis.

6.3. DIAGNOSIS OF TUBERCULOSIS

A complete evaluation for tuberculosis must include medical history and physical examination, chest X-rays, tuberculin skin test, serologic tests and microbiologic smears and cultures. Though a definitive diagnosis of tuberculosis can only be made by culturing *M. tuberculosis* organisms from a specimen taken from the patient, but tuberculosis can be a difficult disease to diagnose, mainly because of the difficulty in culturing the slow-growing *M. tuberculosis* in laboratory [7]. However, the diagnosis of tuberculosis can be based on the guideline of the Diagnostic Standards and Classification of Tuberculosis in Adults and Children. This is an official statement by the American Thoracic Society and the Centers for Disease Control and Prevention [9], which follows the characteristics below:

- Chest X-ray suggestive of tuberculosis opacities;

- Sputum samples that contain acid-fast bacilli on smear microscopy;

- Suggestive histopathologic findings;

- Response to anti-tuberculosis drugs, in individuals with clinical presentation suggestive of tuberculosis.

Signs of tuberculosis activity, or sequel, can be obtained by image methods. Therefore, although in many cases biopsy or culture specimens are required to make the definitive diagnosis, it is imperative that radiologists and clinicians understand the typical distribution, patterns and imaging manifestations of tuberculosis [10]. Chest X-ray in active pulmonary disease can manifest as consolidations, cavitary lesions, reticular/patterns, interstitial (reticulo-nodular), hilar or mediastinal lymphnodemegaly and pleural effusion. Traction bronchiectasis and striations are suggestive of a tuberculosis sequel [3]. This review describes the most common radiographic patterns of pulmonary tuberculosis either with conventional or new methods.

6.4. IMAGE METHODS

6.4.1. Radiography

Although a diagnosis of tuberculosis cannot be established by radiography alone, chest X-ray is a sensitive but nonspecific test to detect tuberculosis. All persons with chest X-ray findings, suggestive of tuberculosis, should have a respiratory specimen submitted for microbiological examination. Radiographic examination of the thorax is useful to identify persons for further evaluation. Confidence in the chest X-ray, as the only diagnostic tool for tuberculosis, will result in an over-diagnosis of tuberculosis while also misdiagnosing tuberculosis and other diseases.

Classically, pulmonary tuberculosis can be divided into primary and post-primary pattern, corresponding to the basic pathogenesis, each presenting with a characteristic radiological presentation. However, it is very difficult to draw distinct lines between those radiographic patterns, while there is considerable overlap in the radiological manifestations [11].

Chest X-ray is the initial image method of choice in the assessment and monitoring pulmonary tuberculosis [3].

6.4.2. Radiological Patterns of Primary Pulmonary Tuberculosis

In primary tuberculosis, a chest X-ray can be normal, although small peripherals nodules can be present, but not be viewed. Lymph node enlargement is the most frequent finding in the primary form of tuberculosis: It affects 83-96% of children although prevalence and incidence decreases with increasing age [7]. Obstructive atelectasis resulting from bronchial extrinsic compression by lymph node enlargement occurs in 9-30% of children with the primary form of the disease [12]. The lymphadenopathy is usually unilateral and located in the hilum or in the paratracheal region [7]. Right paratracheal and hilar localizations are the most common sites of nodal involvement in primary pulmonary tuberculosis, although other combinations have been described (bilateral hilar, isolated mediastinal). Associated parenchymal infiltrates are encountered on the same side as nodal enlargement in approximately two-thirds of pediatric cases of primary pulmonary tuberculosis [11, 13].

Airspace consolidation, usually unilateral, is radiographically evident in approximately 70% of children with primary tuberculosis [7]. Caseous pneumonia represents ganglio-pulmonary tuberculosis, as a result of perforation of an adenopathy in a given bronchus, retro-obstructive pneumonia, and/or atelectasis. It is manifested as segmental or lobar consolidations frequently mimicking typical bacterial pneumonia. Distribution is typically right sided, with obstruction occurring at the right lobar bronchus or bronchus intermedius [3]. Evolution to cavitary disease is rare in children [11]. Inflammation may resorb and evolve to a fibrotic and/or calcified lesion. Destruction and fibrosis of the lung parenchyma result in formation of traction bronchiectasis within the fibrotic region [3].

Primary infection in adults most frequently results in parenchymal consolidation without adenopathy. These infiltrates can excavate leading to phtysis, and according to van Dyck and colleagues (2003) [11] is defined below as:

- Liquefaction of caseous necrosis;

- Formation of cavities;

- Progression to fibrosis and lung destruction.

Also, immunedeficient and elderly patients can present with the childhood type [11].

Miliary tuberculosis refers to extensive dissemination of the disease. It is characterized by diffuse reticulomicronodular opacities arising from hematogenous dissemination of *M. tuberculosis* throw the lung parenchyma; nevertheless, chest X-ray can be normal in 40-50% of cases. It occurs in 2-6% of primary tuberculosis and also occurs in the reactivation of disease [7]. Computed tomography can demonstrate miliary disease before it becomes radiographically apparent. The classic miliary pattern on conventional radiographs is the presence of innumerable micronodular (1 mm) infiltrates, which are all very similar, diffusely scattered in both lungs, especially the lung apices [3; 14]. Thickening of interlobular septa and fine intralobular networks are frequently evident. Diffuse or localized groundglass opacity is sometimes seen [7].

When the primary tuberculosis complex evolves to cure, it can be radiographically evident as a pulmonary nodule or mass, also called tuberculomas, which can be associated with small satellites nodules and/or calcified lymph nodes. The presence of these calcified, satellite, nodules assists the differential diagnosis of solitary pulmonary nodules. Most tuberculomas are less than 3 cm, although lesions greater than 5 cm have been described [3].

The pleural effusion as manifestation of primary tuberculosis occurs in 6-8% of cases [13]. A pulmonary focus can coexist and cannot be easily viewed in the chest X-ray [15]. Pleural effusion is usually on the same side as the primary focus [7]. The presence of suggestive active parenchymal lesions helps diagnosis. The pleural effusion is generally of small to moderate volume [3; 11].

6.4.3. Post-Primary Pulmonary Tuberculosis

Post-primary pulmonary tuberculosis is usually a disease of adults. When observed in the pediatric population it occurs during the adolescence [3]. In the post-primary form, the cavitations are more frequent in the apico-posterior segments of the upper lobes or superior segments of the lower lobes, and occur in 40-45% of cases (Fig. **1**) [7, 12]. Presence of poorly defined nodules and linear opacities can be seen in approximately 25% of patients (Fig. **2**). Tuberculosis reactivation can be manifested as a tuberculoma, defined as a sharply marginated round or oval lesion measuring 0.5-4.0 cm in diameter, in approximately 5% of patient. Satellite nodules around the tuberculoma may be present in as many as 80% of cases [7].

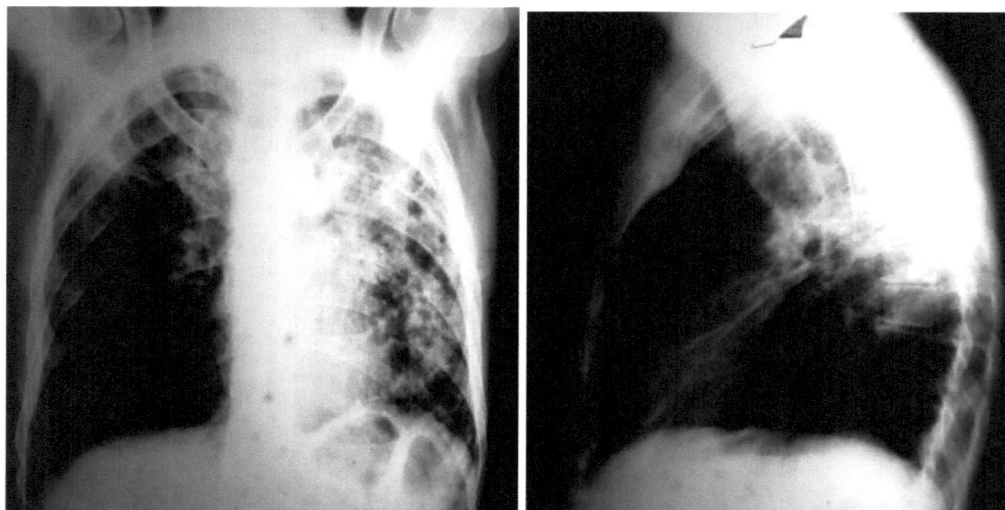

Fig. (1). Chest radiograph showing extensive pulmonary lesions of post-primary pulmonary tuberculosis. Multiple cavitations and fibroproductive lesions in the apical and posterior segments of the right and left lungs is revealed (lateral view). In addition, bronchogenic dissemination is demonstrated. Source: Author.

A suggestive sign of activity is the ipsi- or contra-lateral dissemination, which represents the bronchogenic spreading of *M. tuberculosis* throw lung parenchyma (Fig. **1**). Bronchogenic spread is radiographically identified in 20% of cases of post-primary tuberculosis and manifests as multiple, ill-defined micronodules, distributed in a segmental or lobar pattern, distant from the site of the cavity formation and typically involving the lower lung zones (Fig. **3**). The spread of tuberculosis from a cavity or a lymph node with fistulae also determines reticulo-micronodular opacities [11].

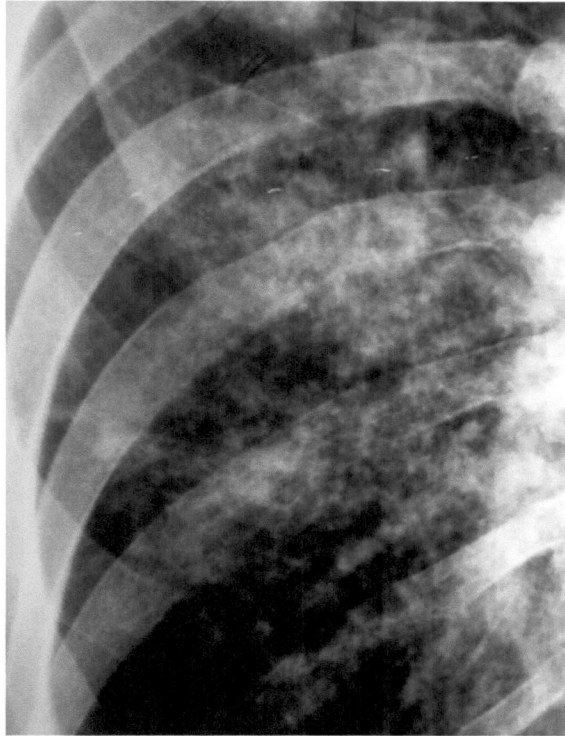

Fig. (2). Parenchymal post-primary tuberculosis. Detail of chest X-ray demonstrates multiple small, centrilobular nodules. Source: Author.

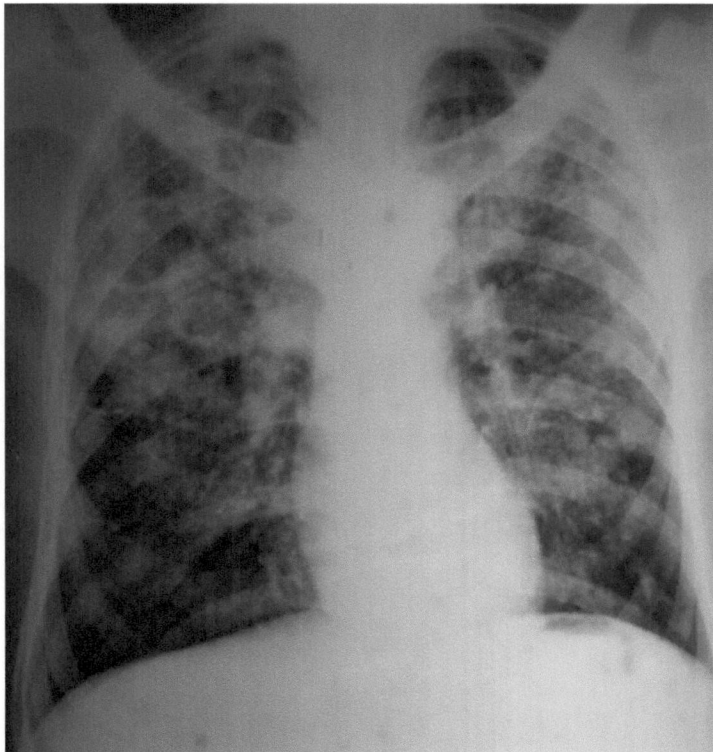

Fig. (3). Bronchogenic spread of post-primary pulmonary tuberculosis. Chest X-ray showing multiple, ill-defined micronodules, distributed bilaterally distant from the site of the cavity formation and involving the lower lung zones. Source: Author.

Hilar or mediastinal lymphadenopathy is uncommon in reactivation of tuberculosis, being seen in approximately 5-10% of patients. Pleural effusion, typically unilateral, occurs in 15-20% of patients (Fig. **4**) [7]. Pleural empyema is uncommon (Fig. **5**).

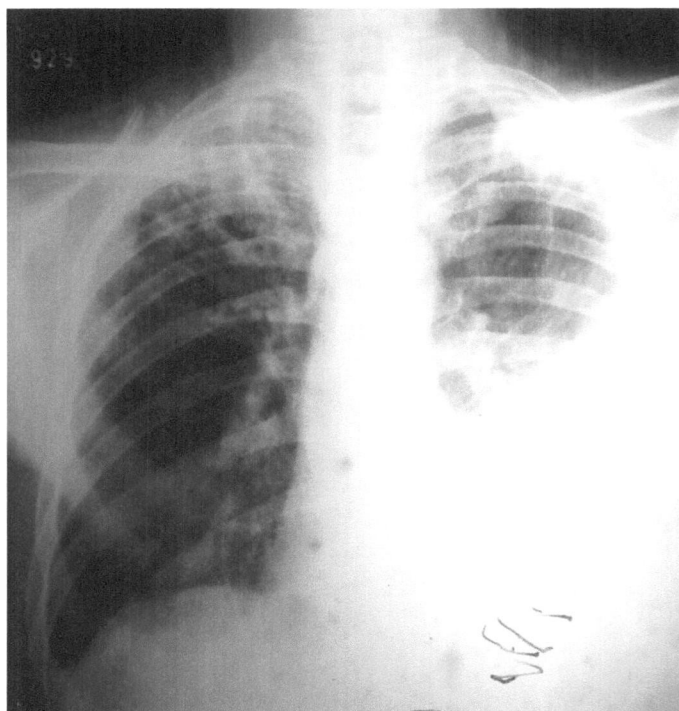

Fig. (4). Post-primary pulmonary tuberculosis. Chest X-ray shows bilateral apical pulmonary infiltration. Note the presence of cavitations on the right upper lobe and associated left sided pleural effusion. Source: Author.

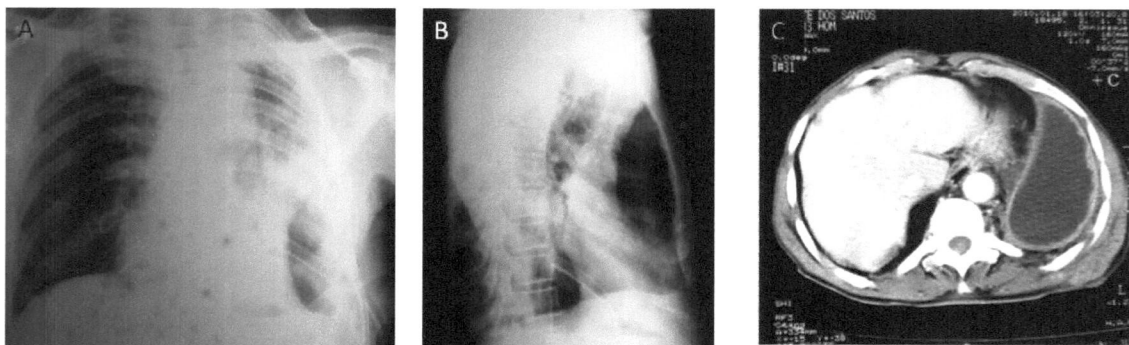

Fig. (5). Pleural empyema secondary to pulmonary tuberculosis. (A and B) Chest X-ray shows a huge cavitation, representing a pneumothorax, and pleural thickening; a drainage tube is observed inside the pleural cavity. (C) Computed tomography demonstrates a thickened pleura and effusion before thoracostomy. Source: Author.

Immunecompromised patients are susceptible to the development of tuberculosis. Known risk factors for development of active disease include conditions that are associated with defects in cell-mediated immunity, such as the ones depicted below:

- HIV infection;

- Malnourished;

- Drug and alcohol abuse;

- Malignancy;

- End-stage renal disease;

- Diabetes mellitus;

- Corticosteroid or other immunosuppressive therapy.

Adalimumab (Humira®), Infliximab (Remicade®) and Etanercept (Enbrel®), mostly used in the treatment of Crohn's disease and rheumatoid arthritis, are humanized antibodies against TNF or its receptor also considered predisposing factors. Unusual or atypical manifestations of pulmonary tuberculosis are common in patients with impaired host immunity. Diabetic and immunecompromised patients have a higher prevalence of multiple cavities and of non-segmental distribution than do patients without underlying disease. Apical cavitations are uncommon in diabetics; however, cavitations in lower segments and involvement of multiple lobes are frequent [16]. Tuberculosis in patients with Systemic Lupus Erythematosus (SLE), tend to show radiologic findings of miliary dissemination, diffuse consolidation, or primary tuberculosis [7].

Chest X-ray manifestations of tuberculosis associated with AIDS depends on the level of immunesuppression and length of illness (Fig. **6**). Among severe immunecompromised patients co-infected with *M. tuberculosis* and HIV, 10-20% have normal chest X-rays [17], or show similar findings of those with primary tuberculosis, including lymphadenopathy and pleural effusion. The more frequent radiological findings are miliary spread and diffuse consolidations.

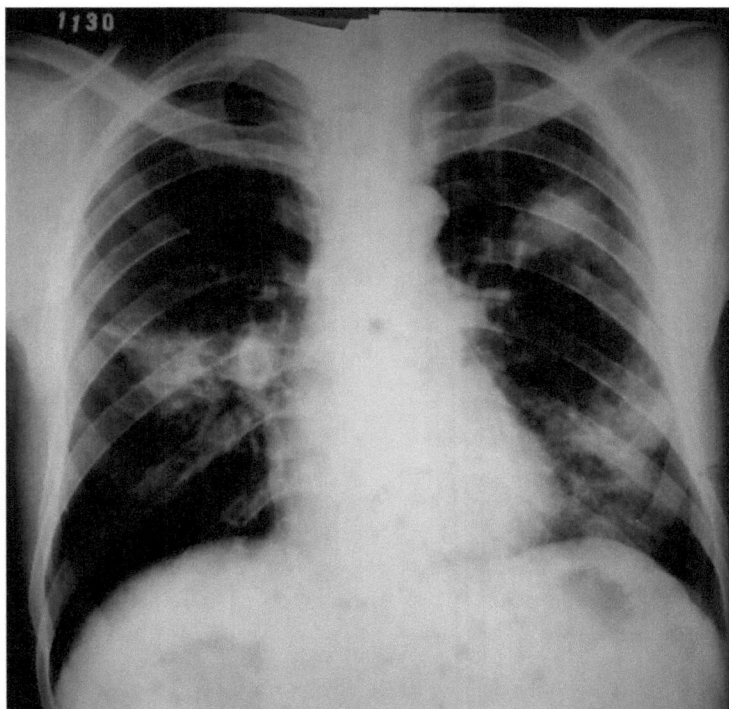

Fig. (6). Unusual manifestations of pulmonary tuberculosis in male patient with AIDS. Irregular consolidations distributed in lower lobes and left superior lobe. Source: Author.

Parenchymal changes can be focal (alveolar opacities) or diffuse, with miliar prevalence. Atypical presentations are common in elderly people, diabetes mellitus and patients with SLE (due to impairment of cellular immunity and exposition to high doses of corticosteroids). Cavitations, calcifications, and fibrosis are infrequent in patient with AIDS [18]. These changes are more common in lower lobes.

Parenchymal striations, calcifications, and retraction can be a result of cure. Thin wall cavities may also remain after cure, representing the sequel of the process [19]. Up to 40% of patients with post-primary tuberculosis have a marked fibrotic response, this manifests as atelectasis of the upper lobe, retraction of hilum, compensatory lower lobe hyperinflation, and mediastinal shift towards the fibrotic lung. Apical pleural thickening associated with fibrosis may reveal proliferation of extrapleural fatty tissue and peripheral atelectasis on regular tomography. Complete destruction of a whole lung or a major part of a lung is not uncommon at the end stage of pulmonary tuberculosis (Fig. **7**) [3, 11, 20].

In addition, those typical aspects of the chest X-ray in children can also be found and compared in the append section.

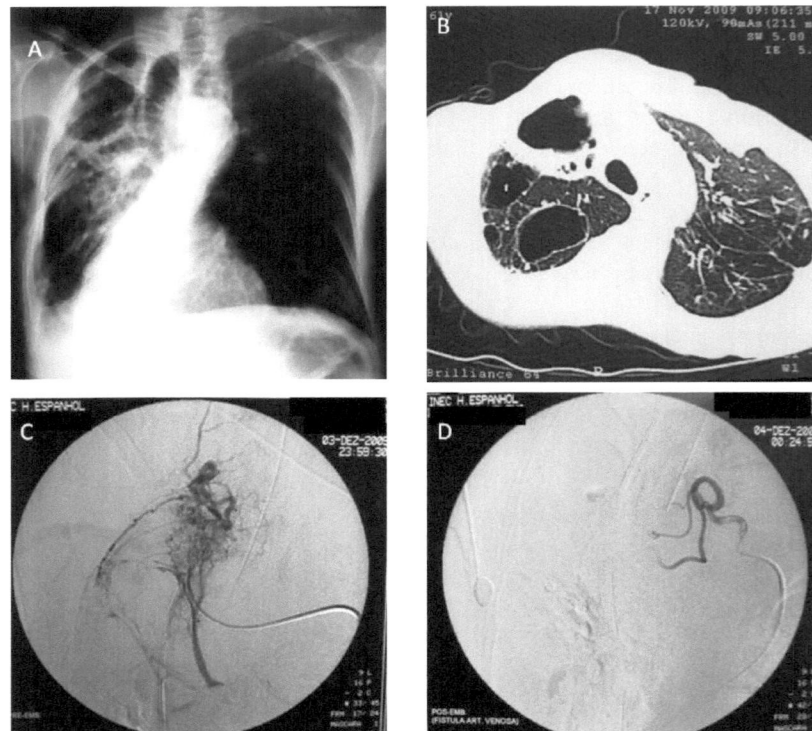

Fig. (7). Extensive pulmonary sequelae of past treated tuberculosis in a 57-years old woman, with severe hemoptysis. (A) Chest X-ray shows destruction of right upper lobe, homolateral tracheal deviation, pleural thickening, and scoliosis. (B) High-resolution computed tomography, obtained at level of aortic arch, shows destruction of the right upper lobe, with multiple bronchiectasis and huge cavities. Note also satellite lesion with parenchymal distortion in the left upper lobe. (C) Arteriography showing vascular lush bed, presence of pseudo-aneurysms and fistulas in the bronchial artery branches and tirobicervico-scapular trunk. (D) After embolization with polyvinyl alcohol (PVA) particles, arteriography shows vascular exclusion. Source: Author.

6.4.4. Computed Tomography

The chest computed tomography (CT) is a method used in clinical suspicion of pulmonary tuberculosis, especially in cases where the initial X-ray is normal. Chest CT is superior to chest X-ray in the initial assessment of tuberculosis [21-24]. CT is more sensitive than chest radiography in the detection and characterization of both slight localized or disseminated parenchymal disease and mediastinal lymphadenopathy [7]. It is an aid in differentiation from other chest diseases, especially in patients with AIDS or fever of unknown etiology and when there is disagreement between the clinical findings and chest X-ray. High-resolution chest CT is extremely accurate in tuberculosis diagnosis [24]. With CT, the diagnosis of pulmonary tuberculosis is correct in 91% of patients and is correctly excluded in 76% of patients [7]. Despite the high accuracy of CT, sputum smears has superior specificity and must be included in the initial assessment [3].

Thorax CT is more effective in assessing the extent of parenchymal disease, although the chest X-ray is an efficient diagnostic method to discover the tuberculosis illness activity [3]. CT scanning is considered the modality of choice for lymph node detection in the chest. The disadvantages include (i) limited availability, (ii) high radiation dose and (iii) the need for intravenous contrast medium [25].

Tuberculous Adenopathies, a form of primary tuberculosis, often measures more than 2 cm and shows a very characteristic, but not pathognomonic, "rim sign". It consists of a low-density center (representing caseous necrosis), surrounded by a peripheral enhancing rim. On contrast-enhanced CT scans, this rim represents the vascular rim of the granulomatous inflammatory tissue [26]. This "rim sign" has also been found with atypical mycobacteria, lymphoma [27], and testis carcinoma [28]. Parenchymal opacities are typically located in the periphery of the lung, especially in the subpleural areas. They are difficult to see on conventional radiographs; therefore, CT is often necessary to detect these slight parenchymal infiltrates [11]. On CT, parenchymal consolidation in primary tuberculosis is most commonly dense and homogeneous, but may also be patchy, linear, nodular, or mass-like [7].

The presence of cavities is an important sign of active tuberculosis disease. Frequently, high resolution CT demonstrates small cavities surrounded by consolidations that are not seen on ordinary chest X-rays. Thick walled cavities are observed in up to 76% of patients with pulmonary tuberculosis in the occasion of its diagnosis [24].

Segmentar centrilobular nodules, representing bronchogenic dissemination, are the most common CT finding in active disease (82-100%). It is represented as multiple, ill-defined micronodules, dispersed in a segmental or lobar distribution, distant from the site of the cavity formation and typically involving the lower lung zones [11]. These nodules frequently conflate in 62-71%, or form larger nodules in almost 66% of the cases. Segmental or lobar consolidation is observed in 47-62% of cases and may be associated with hilar or mediastinal lymphnodemegaly [3]. High-resolution CT is the imaging technique of choice to reveal early bronchogenic spread [21]. The typical findings are 2-4 mm centrilobular nodules and are sharply marginated linear branching opacities (tree-in-bud sign). These have been shown to represent the endobronchial spread and are due to caseous necrosis containing bacilli within and around terminal and respiratory bronchioles [7, 11].

The bronchial wall thickening occurs in approximately 62% of cases and bronchiectasis is observed in 23% of patients with active pulmonary tuberculosis. The aspect "tree-in-bud" or bronchiolar thickening is presented in up to 57% of cases [3, 24]. Local emphysema can be present as result of architecture distortion [3]. Coexistence of low and high-density areas is recognized as mosaic appearance, as a result of air trapping secondary to constrictive bronchiolitis. Thin walled cavities are seen in 21%, traction bronchiectasis in 86%, and bands are found 77% of treated patients [3, 21, 24]. Thin-walled cavities, traction bronchiectasis and bands are found in 21%, 86% and 77% of treated patients, respectively [3, 21, 24].

Miliary tuberculosis at thin-section CT shows a mixture of both sharply and poorly defined, 1-4 mm nodules, in a diffuse, random distribution often associated with intra- and inter-lobular septal thickening [12]. The more widespread location of these micronodules, including subpleural location, excludes the diagnosis of lymphangitis carcinomatose and bronchiolitis [29].

Tuberculosis can involve airways in 10-20% of all patients with pulmonary disease. Central airways are more frequently affected. This is the most common cause of inflammatory stricture of the bronchus indeed. The principal CT findings of tracheobronchial tuberculosis are circumferential wall thickening and luminal narrowing, with involvement of a long segment of the bronchi. In active disease, the airways are irregularly narrowed in their lumina and have thick walls; whereas, in fibrotic disease, the airways are smoothly narrowed and usually have thin walls [7].

On CT, lower prevalence of cavitation, higher prevalence of mediastinal or hilar lymphadenopathy, and often extrapulmonary involvement are observed in HIV-seropositive patients with a CD4 T lymphocyte count lower than 200/mm^3. This is compared with HIV-seropositive patients with a CD4 T lymphocyte count equal to, or higher than 200/mm³. Severe immunesuppression is also associated with miliary or disseminated disease [7]. For simply comparison to chest X-ray infant case, a typical CT scan result can be found in the append section as well.

6.4.5. Nuclear Medicine

Images obtained through nuclear medicine result from functional or metabolic changes detected of the emission of gamma rays from certain radiopharmaceutical dyes. Tuberculosis diagnosis can become difficult in children when based on; positive sputum samples, X-ray changes, tomographic findings, HIV immunecompromised individuals, tuberculosis sequel, or suspected reactivation. In these situations, metabolic or functional studies provide tools for diagnosis and monitoring tuberculosis [3].

6.4.6. Gallium-67-Citrate Scintigraphy

Gallium-67-citrate scintigraphy is a useful supplementary method in the assessment of infectious diseases, including pulmonary tuberculosis, especially in imunessupressed patients. Increased cavity can be observed in most patients with active tuberculosis, while it is always negative in patients with inactive, latent disease [3]. Gallium-67-citrate scintigraphy has high sensitivity in identifying extrapulmonary tuberculosis [10]. In patients with AIDS, gallium-67-citrate scintigraphy is more sensitive than other imaging methods in infectious site location. However, the specificity is low in evaluating pulmonary tuberculosis due to the high incidence of other opportunistic infections. The combination of radiography and gallium-67-citrate scintigraphy increases sensitivity for discovery early tuberculosis, although confirmation by other methods is required [30]. The gallium-67 compound is a marker of inflammatory reaction, i.e. captured in infectious or inflammatory processes and fundamentally depending on increased capillary permeability. The cavity can remain increased after pulmonary tuberculosis treatment as result of persistent inflammatory process [3].

6.4.7. Inhalation and Perfusion Pulmonary Scintigraphy

Inhalation and perfusion pulmonary scintigraphy performed with technetium-99m compound may have a complementary role in initial assessment and pulmonary tuberculosis follow-up [31]. The method can assess the extent of lung damage. Inhalation/perfusion scan studies, associated with functional respiratory tests and chest CT, confer information on the degree of lung damage and can help the pre-operatory evaluation of surgical treatment of pulmonary sequel and multidrug-resistant pulmonary tuberculosis [3].

6.4.8. Positrons Emission Tomography

The positrons emission tomography (PET) is a non-invasive method whose basic principle is the use of marked biological compounds with high atomic instability elements which are positrons transmitters (particles with the same mass of electron, but with opposite charge). This method allows the glucose metabolism (fluorodeoxyglucose, or FDG) study and is useful in the differentiation of benign from malignant lesions [3].

Based on Burrill and colleagues (2007) [10], FDG PET has several advantages over gallium and indium scanning, as depicted below:

- It can be performed immediately, with no delay required between injection and scanning.

- It generally results in a lower radiation dose due to the short half-life of FDG.

- It demonstrates little normal organ uptake, except in the brain and heart.

- It provides a quantitative measurement of the absolute fraction of the injected dose reaching a tissue.

Due to active glucose metabolism, caused by active granulomatous inflammation, tuberculomas have sometimes been reported to accumulate FDG and to cause PET scans to be interpreted as false-positives for malignancy. FDG PET detects inflammation that occurs in active tuberculosis disease and that may persist, at lower intensity, after the treatment. This method is image-based, and thus an important resource for the diagnosis and monitoring of pulmonary tuberculosis [3, 7].

Increased caption FDG has been verified in both pulmonary and ganglionary tuberculosis [3, 32]. Detecting signs of tuberculosis activity makes image methods important subsidies for the diagnosis of pulmonary disease, especially when the sputum smear confirmation or culture is not possible. However, increased uptake is also seen with other granulomatous diseases and infections such as sarcoidosis, histoplasmosis, aspergillosis, and coccidioidomycosis [10].

PET CT for the evaluation and follow-up of solitary pulmonary nodule and non-small cell lung cancer can provide additional useful information to conventional radiology for treatment planning and a non-invasive determination of prognosis. However, physicians need to be aware of the limitations of this imaging modality, particularly when tuberculosis has a high prevalence in the population [33]. Therefore, in the setting of a known pulmonary lesion, FGD PET cannot be used to differentiate between neoplasic and non-neoplasic causes [10]. However, 11C-choline PET scans can help to differentiate between lung cancer and tuberculoma. The standard uptake value of tuberculoma is low in 11C-choline PET scans [7].

6.5. RADIOLOGIC FINDINGS OF THORACIC TUBERCULOSIS IN CHILDREN

Despite specificity, the chest roentgenogram remains the most used diagnostic test in clinical practice. Latent tuberculosis infection can be diagnosed as a calcified lesion (old granuloma), found in lungs fields as well as a positive tuberculin skin test or *in vitro* assay (IGRA). The mediastinal lymph gland enlargement is most commonly seen in the hilar regions of the lung (Fig. **8**). The lymph gland enlargement is usually unilateral, but bilateral lymph gland enlargement does occur [34, 35]. Hilar or mediastinal lymphadenopathy is the most common radiological feature found in children with tuberculosis (Fig. **8**). Hilar lymphadenopathy is best seen on a posteroanterior radiograph as a lobulated density, but can also be viewed in lateral films posterior to the bronchus intermedius.

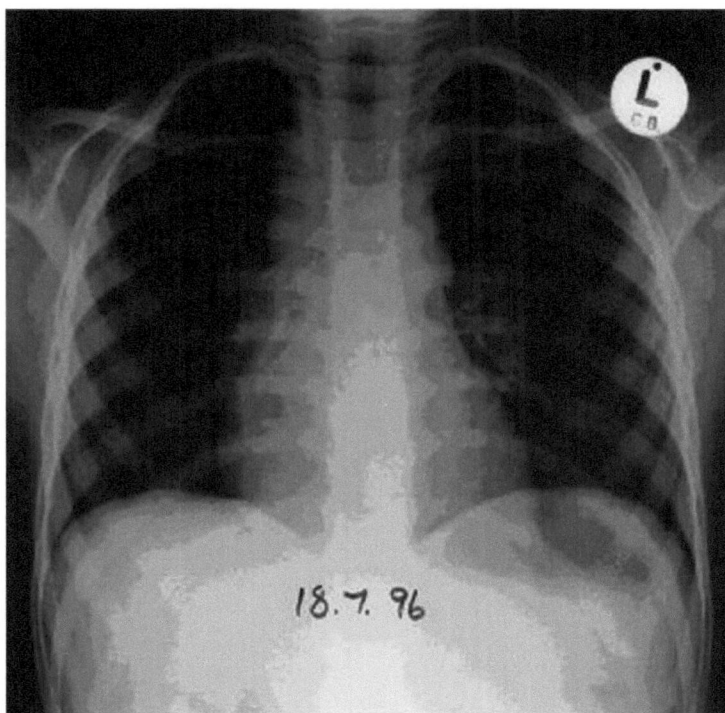

Fig. (8). Suspected hilar and paratracheal lymph gland enlargement. Source: Reproduced with permission of the copyright owner: Robert Gie. International Union Against Tuberculosis and Lung Disease.

Parenchymal infiltrates are encountered on the same side as nodal enlargement in approximately two-thirds of pediatric cases of primary pulmonary tuberculosis (Fig. **9**).

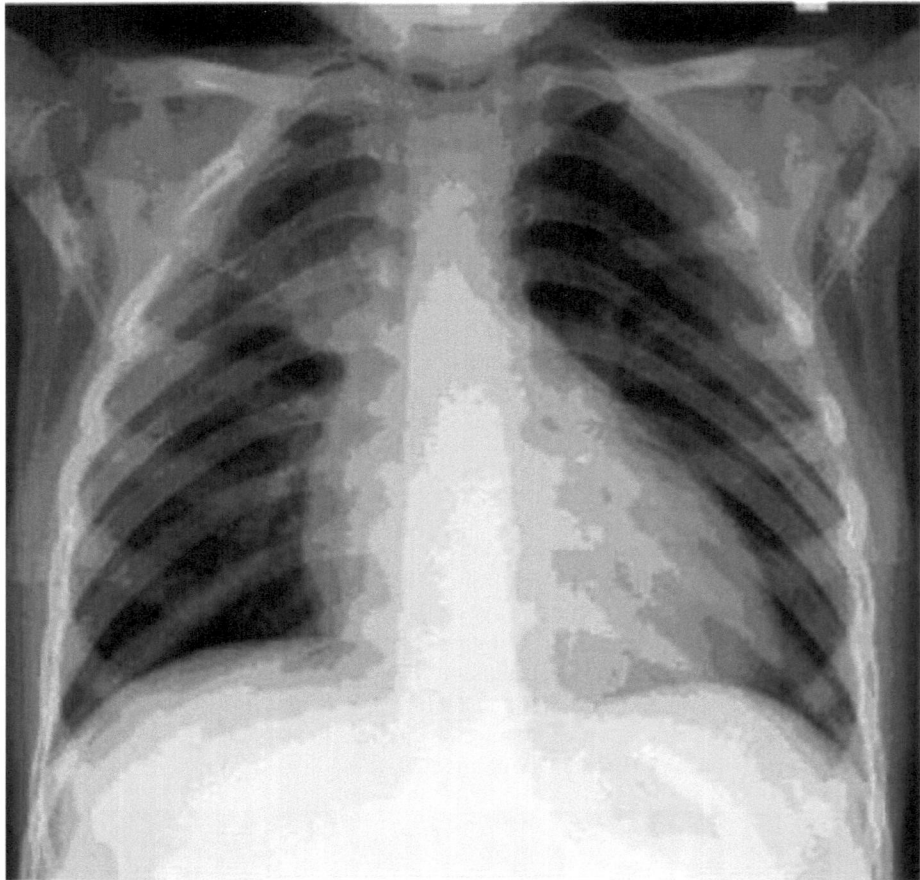

Fig. (9). Hilar lymph node enlargement with infiltration into the surrounding lung tissue. Source: Reproduced with permission of the copyright owner: Robert Gie. International Union Against Tuberculosis and Lung Disease.

Massive paratracheal lymph gland enlargement without visible hilar lymph gland enlargement seldom occurs [34]. Frequently, the hilar lymph node enlargement is not distinguishable from the pulmonary vessels. In this case, careful evaluation of the airways is often helpful, as compression of the airways, especially the right and left main bronchi, is indirect evidence of hilar lymph gland enlargement. However, airway compression due to lymph node enlargement is more common in younger. A more penetrated chest X-ray is often useful for visualizing the airways (Fig. **10**).

Occasionally, the involved lymph nodes obstruct the bronchi, causing a clinical picture that is often confused with asthma. An uncommon finding is the unilateral hyperinflation secondary to incomplete obstruction of the central bronchi, where the narrowing acts as a "check valve", allowing air to be trapped in the affected lobe or lung (Fig. **11**) [34].

Alveolar consolidation can occur as a result of lymph node ulceration through the bronchus wall, causing occlusion of the bronchus as well as aspiration of infected material into the lobe. The immunological response in the lobe leads to the accumulation of infected material. This process leads to expansion in the size of the lobe. The increase in size of the lobe is seen by upward or downward displacement of the fissures [34; 35]. Atelectasis of a segment, or lobe, occurs as a result of complete obstruction of an airway by the infected lymph node. The lobes affected are usually the right middle lobe or the lower lobes.

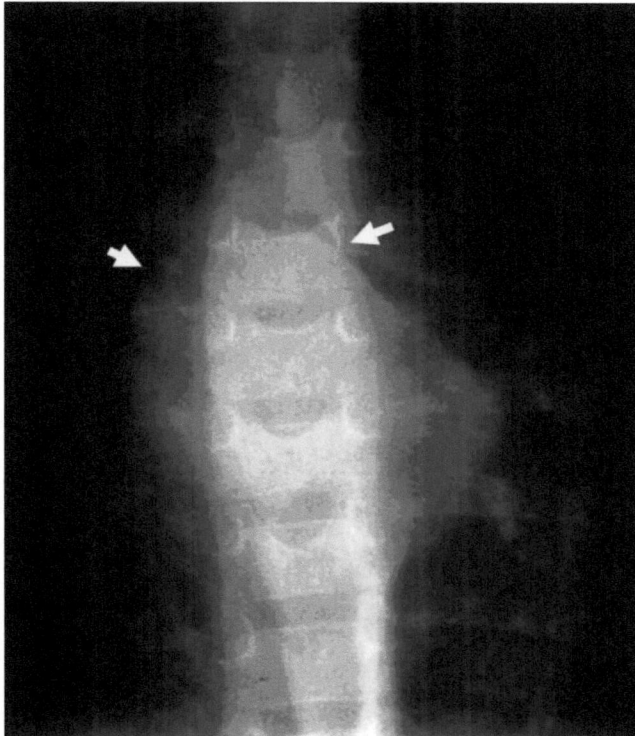

Fig. (10). Compression of the large subcarinal lymph nodes airways (see arrows). Source: Reproduced with permission of the copyright owner: Robert Gie. International Union Against Tuberculosis and Lung Disease.

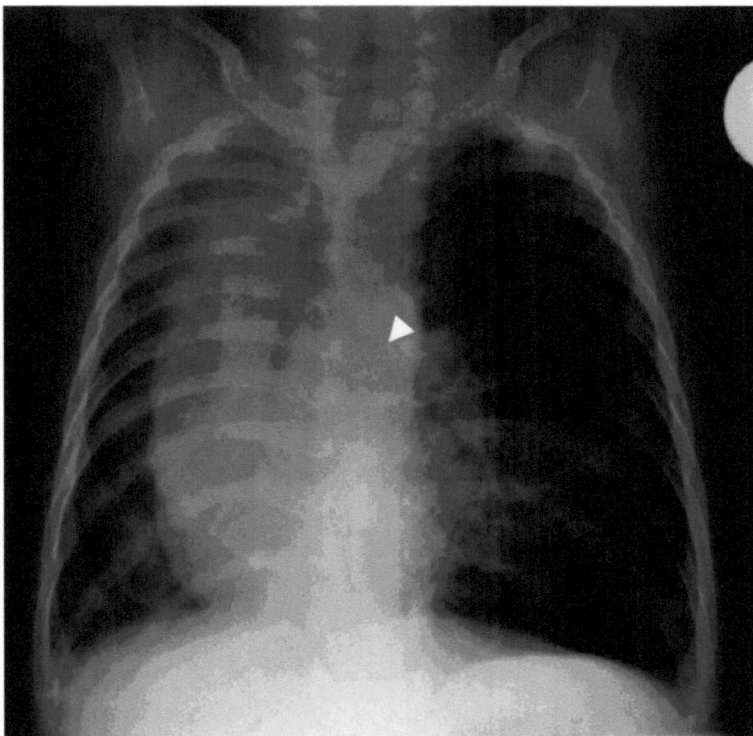

Fig. (11). The left main bronchus partially obstructed, acting as a "check valve" leading to hyperinflation of the left lung (see arrow head). Source: Reproduced with permission of the copyright owner: Robert Gie. International Union Against Tuberculosis and Lung Disease.

Diffuse fine bilateralreticular shadowing, sometimes called a snowstorm appearance, is typical of miliary tuberculosis. Miliary tuberculosis is secondary to hematogenous dissemination of a large number of organisms following the involvement of blood vessels by the primary complex. These large numbers of bacilli are then spread throughout the body and lead to the development of granulomas in all the involved organs. The granulomas are all similar in size, they are seen on chest radiographs as evenly distributed, small (less than 2 mm), round opacities (Fig. **12**). They are best observed on chest X-rays in the lower lobes [34], while occasionally a focal mass can be seen [35].

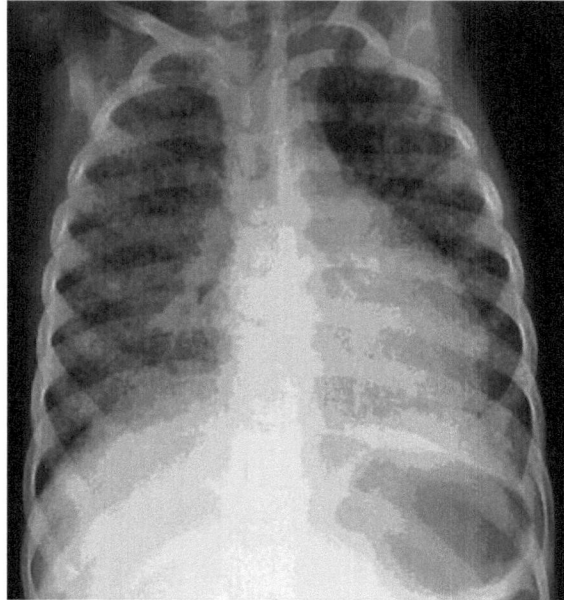

Fig. (12). Fine millet-sized nodules typically seen in miliary tuberculosis. The nodules are all of similar size and spread through the lung fields. Source: Reproduced with permission of the copyright owner: Robert Gie. International Union Against Tuberculosis and Lung Disease.

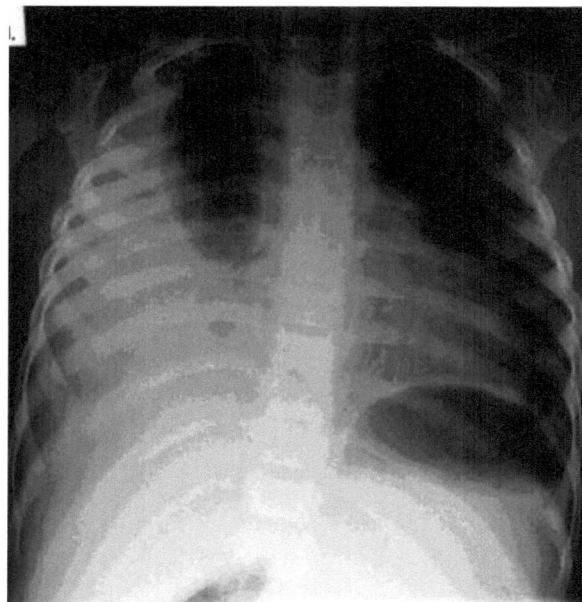

Fig. (13). Uncomplicated right sided pleural effusion with no other radiological signs of primary tuberculosis visible. Source: Reproduced with permission of the copyright owner: Robert Gie. International Union Against Tuberculosis and Lung Disease.

Adolescents can present with adult-type reactivation disease. Pleural tuberculosis is also more commonly seen in teenagers than in younger children (Fig. **13**). Tuberculosis is the most common cause for a large pleural effusion in an adolescent patient [34]. Contrast enhanced CT imaging can be helpful. Tuberculosis adenopathies often show the presence of conglomerated nodal masses with central lucency. Particular manifestations, such as endobronchial involvement, bronchiectasis, and early cavitation are more apparent on CT imaging than chest X-rays. CT imaging is also useful in demonstrating pleural or pericardial disease. The use of magnetic resonance imaging for demonstrating intrathoracic lymphadenopathy is limited because of the sedation and respiratory gating requirements [35].

6.6. CONCLUDING REMARKS

Chest X-ray films are still the first image method in evaluating suspected pulmonary tuberculosis in children and adults. The CT scan has some impact on patient management, and while the CT evaluation may be helpful in determination of disease activity in some patients, definitive diagnosis requires isolation and identification of *M. tuberculosis* species from clinical specimens. Nuclear image methods are alternative resources, which can help discriminate active from past TB. Specially, in children, the diagnosis of tuberculosis must be based on the history of contact with an adult index case, symptoms and signs, tuberculin skin test or IGRA, chest X-rays, scoring systems and diagnostic algorithms.

REFERENCES

[1]   Wong VS, Tan SY. Wilhelm Conrad Rontgen (1845-1923): a light in the dark. Singapore Med J 2009; 50(9): 851-2.

[2]   Singh SP, Nath H. Early radiology of pulmonary tuberculosis. AJR Am J Roentgenol 1994; 162(4): 846.

[3]   Bombarda S, Figueiredo CL, Funari MNG, Soares J·nior J, Seiscento M, Terra Filho M. Imagem em tuberculose pulmonar. J Pneumol 2001; 27(6): 329-40.

[4]   Murray JF. A century of tuberculosis. Am J Respir Crit Care Med 2004; 169(11): 1181-6.

[5]   Pratt PC. Pathology of tuberculosis. Semin Roentgenol 1979; 14(3): 196-203.

[6]   Russell DG, Cardona PJ, Kim MJ, Allain S, Altare F. Foamy macrophages and the progression of the human tuberculosis granuloma. Nat Immunol 2009; 10(9): 943-8.

[7]   Jeong YJ, Lee KS. Pulmonary tuberculosis: up-to-date imaging and management. AJR Am J Roentgenol 2008; 191(3): 834-44.

[8]   Ehlers S. Lazy,dynamic or minimally recrudescent? On the elusive nature and location of the *Mycobacterium* responsible for latent tuberculosis. Infection 2009; 37(2): 87-95.

[9]   American Thoracic Society, Centers for Disease Control and Prevention. Diagnostic standards and classification of tuberculosis in adults and children. Am J Respir Crit Care Med; 2000. Report No. 161.

[10]   Burrill J, Williams CJ, Bain G, Conder G, Hine AL, Misra RR. Tuberculosis: a radiologic review. Radiographics 2007; 27(5): 1255-73.

[11]   van Dyck P, Vanhoenacker FM, van den Brande P, De Schepper AM. Imaging of pulmonary tuberculosis. Eur Radiol 2003; 13(8): 1771-85.

[12]   Leung AN. Pulmonary tuberculosis: the essentials. Radiology 1999; 210(2): 307-22.

[13]   Leung AN, Muller NL, Pineda PR, FitzGerald JM. Primary tuberculosis in childhood: radiographic manifestations. Radiology 1992; 182(1): 87-91.

[14]   Kwong JS, Carignan S, Kang EY, Muller NL, FitzGerald JM. Miliary tuberculosis: Diagnostic accuracy of chest radiography. Chest 1996; 110(2): 339-42.

[15]   Choyke PL, Sostman HD, Curtis AM, *et al.* Adult-onset pulmonary tuberculosis. Radiology 1983; 148(2): 357-62.

[16]   Perez-Guzman C, Torres-Cruz A, Villarreal-Velarde H, Vargas MH. Progressive age-related changes in pulmonary tuberculosis images and the effect of diabetes. Am J Respir Crit Care Med 2000; 162(5): 1738-40.

[17]   Greenberg SD, Frager D, Suster B, Walker S, Stavropoulos C, Rothpearl A. Active pulmonary tuberculosis in patients with AIDS: spectrum of radiographic findings including a normal appearance. Radiology 1994; 193(1): 115-9.

[18]   Marchiori E, As S. Manifestacoes tadiologicas pulmonares nos portadores da sindrome da imunodeficiencia adquirida. J Pneumol 1999; 25: 167-5.

[19] Miller WT, MacGregor RR. Tuberculosis: frequency of unusual radiographic findings. AJR Am J Roentgenol 1978; 130(5): 867-75.

[20] Im JG, Webb WR, Han MC, Park JH. Apical opacity associated with pulmonary tuberculosis: high-resolution CT findings. Radiology 1991; 178(3): 727-31.

[21] Im JG, Itoh H, Shim YS, *et al.* Pulmonary tuberculosis: CT findings-early active disease and sequential change with antituberculous therapy. Radiology 1993; 186(3): 653-60.

[22] Lee KS, Im JG. CT in adults with tuberculosis of the chest: characteristic findings and role in management. AJR Am J Roentgenol 1995; 164(6): 1361-7.

[23] Hatipoglu ON, Osma E, Manisali M, *et al.* High resolution computed tomographic findings in pulmonary tuberculosis. Thorax 1996; 51(4): 397-402.

[24] Lee KS, Hwang JW, Chung MP, Kim H, Kwon OJ. Utility of CT in the evaluation of pulmonary tuberculosis in patients without AIDS. Chest 1996; 110(4): 977-84.

[25] Andronikou S, Wieselthaler N. Modern imaging of tuberculosis in children: thoracic,central nervous system and abdominal tuberculosis. Pediatr Radiol 2004; 34(11): 861-75.

[26] Kim WS, Moon WK, Kim IO, *et al.* Pulmonary tuberculosis in children: evaluation with CT. AJR Am. J Roentgenol 1997; 168(4): 1005-9.

[27] Im JG, Song KS, Kang HS, *et al.* Mediastinal tuberculous lymphadenitis: CT manifestations. Radiology 1987; 164(1): 115-9.

[28] Woodring JH, Vandiviere HM, Fried AM, Dillon ML, Williams TD, Melvin IG. Update: the radiographic features of pulmonary tuberculosis. AJR Am J Roentgenol 1986; 146(3): 497-506.

[29] Webb WR, Muller NL, Naidich DP. Diseases characterized primarily by nodular or reticulonodular opacities. In: Webb WR, Muller NL, Naidich DP, editors. High-resolution CT of the lung. Lippincott Williams and Wilkins. Philadelphia 2001.

[30] Abdel-Dayem HM, Naddaf S, Aziz M, *et al.* Sites of tuberculous involvement in patients with AIDS: Autopsy findings and evaluation of gallium imaging. Clin Nucl Med 1997; 22(5): 310-4.

[31] Degirmenci B, Kilinc O, Cirak KA, *et al.* Technetium-99m-tetrofosmin scintigraphy in pulmonary tuberculosis. J Nucl Med 1998; 39(12): 2116-20.

[32] Bakheet SM, Powe J, Ezzat A, Rostom A. F-18-FDG uptake in tuberculosis. Clin Nucl Med 1998; 23(11): 739-42.

[33] Low SY, Eng P, Keng GH, Ng DC. Positron emission tomography with CT in the evaluation of non-small cell lung cancer in populations with a high prevalence of tuberculosis. Respirology 2006; 11(1): 84-9.

[34] Gie R. Diagnostic atlas of intrathoracic tuberculosis in children: A guide for low income countries. International Union Against Tuberculosis and Lung Disease. France 2003.

[35] Lighter J, Rigaud M. Diagnosing childhood tuberculosis: traditional and innovative modalities. Curr Probl Pediatr Adolesc Health Care 2009; 3 9: 61-88.

CHAPTER 7

New Laboratory Techniques for the Diagnosis of Tuberculosis

Theolis Barbosa[1,*] and Paulo R.Z. Antas[2]

[1]*Laboratório Integrado de Microbiologia e Imunoregulação, Centro de Pesquisa Gonçalo Moniz, Fiocruz, Rua Waldemar Falcão, # 121, Candeal; zip: 40296-710, Salvador, Bahia, Brazil and* [2]*Laboratório de Imunologia Clínica, Fiocruz, Av. Brasil, # 4365; zip: 21045-900, Rio de Janeiro, Brazil*

Abstract: New diagnostic tools for active and latent tuberculosis have been proposed in the last decades, but real progress in disease management is still lacking. Many recent reviews have addressed the subject, with special interest in comparing the performance of the different methods. In this chapter, some of the new strategies that are currently in the market will be discussed. Presented will be the principles underlying those strategies, and stress their present value in the diagnosis of pediatric tuberculosis disease. Combining methods maybe necessary to address the diagnosis of tuberculosis in its multiplicity of forms, while the testing of different combinations might yield promising diagnostic trees that could be used with the necessary accuracy and reproducibility in the field.

Keywords: Tuberculosis Control, Early Diagnosis, Treatment Decision, Children.

7.1. BACKGROUND

Tuberculosis is a multifaceted disease. Although, in most cases, the affected organ is the lung, in approximately 30% of the cases the disease occurs in extrapulmonary sites: such as the lymph nodes, the pleura, the pericardium, the peritoneum, the central nervous system, the liver, the intestine, the genito-urinary tract, the eyes, the joints and bones, and the skin. All this can be in combination, or not, with lung disease [1, 2]. Involvement of extrapulmonary sites is seen more frequently in children and in immunecompromised patients [1]. Disease is, however, not manifested in most of the individuals infected with the etiologic agent, *Mycobacterium tuberculosis*. In these individuals, bacilli are contained by the immune response and the individual presents a latent or dormant, asymptomatic form of the disease. These are assessable only by tests of the immunological response against specific *M. tuberculosis* antigens, or by demonstration of calcified lung foci representing healed lesions by imaging techniques (see chapter 6).

The clinical diagnosis of tuberculosis is based on a positive tuberculin skin test (TST) response, clinical and radiological signs and symptoms compatible with the disease, and response to treatment. Laboratory confirmation, considered the gold-standard for case definition, is achieved by demonstration of acid-fast bacilli (AFB) and/or culture and microbiological identification of *M. tuberculosis* from a relevant clinical specimen. The U.S.A. Centers for Disease Control and Prevention (CDC) also consider the amplification of mycobacterial nucleic acids and a positive response in the *in vitro* assay (IGRA) using approved tests as auxiliary in disease diagnostics [2; 3]. Not all of these methodologies may be available, especially in limited-resource settings. The importance of a fast tuberculosis diagnosis is underlined by the fact that, if left untreated, diseased individuals can be highly infectious, and potential non-household contacts can be hard to trace, this is due to tuberculosis being an airborne disease.

Visualization of bacilli in sputum smears is achieved at best in up to 50-70% of clinical samples. Lower detection rates are achieved for populations with a high proportion of tuberculosis and HIV co-infected patients [4-6]. Negative sputum samples are usually submitted to culture, to check for mycobacterial growth, and with this it is possible to detect up to 80% of true tuberculosis cases [4, 7]. However, culture is

---

*Address correspondence to Theolis Barbosa: Laboratório Integrado de Microbiologia e Imunoregulação, Centro de Pesquisa Gonçalo Moniz, Fiocruz, Rua Waldemar Falcão, # 121, Candeal; zip: 40296-710, Salvador, Bahia, Brazil; Tel: +55 71 3176-2259; Fax: +55 71 3176-2279; E-mail: theolis@bahia.fiocruz.br

often not available in low-income settings, due to lack of infrastructure and trained personnel [8], as well as its sensitivity is highly variable among different laboratories [1]. Classically, cultures are performed in solid medium, where *M. tuberculosis* growth is achieved only within 6-8 weeks [1]. Thus, for smear-negative cases, treatment is often initiated on the basis of clinical, radiological and other laboratory-based findings [4]. Moreover, empirical management can be used simply based on an algorithm approach.

Children under 10 years-old are especially difficult to diagnose, as they are less likely to present the sputum-positive form of pulmonary tuberculosis. In children, cavity lung disease is much less frequent; therefore, they expectorate sputum less frequently. This, in turn, makes the bacteriological confirmation of pediatric cases a difficult task [9]. Differential diagnosis of pulmonary tuberculosis by non-microbiological methods is also more difficult, as many child diseases present clinical and radiological features similar to those found in tuberculosis adult cases, especially among M. tuberculosis and HIV co-infected or malnourished populations [1]. Extrapulmonary disease, especially tuberculous lymphadenitis and meningitis, also occurs much more often in children than in adults [7]. M. tuberculosis can be recovered in up to 60% of cases from pus, aspirates or biopsies of lymph nodes in children with suspected disease. Culture of lymph node biopsy samples increases the detection rate to 90%, but involves more invasive procedures [1]. Finally, latently infected children have a higher risk of progression to active form of tuberculosis, and constitute an important reservoir of future disease in the adulthood [9]. From an epidemiological perspective, the investigation of household contacts of adult pulmonary tuberculosis index cases is of utmost importance to control pediatric tuberculosis, as half of asymptomatic children in contact with a pulmonary tuberculosis patient present abnormal chest X-ray findings [7]. Furthermore, the frequency of pediatric cases is much increased in high burden settings [9].

New, more accurate and faster laboratory diagnosis methods are needed to aid in tuberculosis control worldwide, and research in the field has yielded novel tests that have been made available in the market in the last decades. In this chapter, we discuss some of these tests, emphasizing those currently offered "off the shelf", and the results that have been obtained with their application, especially focusing on the diagnosis of pediatric tuberculosis.

7.2. BACTERIOLOGICAL

7.2.1. Improved Visualization of Bacilli in Smears

The Ziehl-Neelsen stained smears (or AFB, for acid-fast bacilli) are the current gold-standard for direct observation of mycobacteria in clinical specimens. The positivity of sputum smears from pediatric patients is very low, around 10-15%, even though sputum smears are considered of diagnostic value for children above 10 years of age. The fluorescent Auramine O (AuO) dye has been used as a substitute for classical AFB staining to help visualization of bacilli. AuO allows improved sensitivity and reduced time of reading per slide, but the need for expensive fluorescence microscopes has been an obstacle to the implementation of this technique (reviewed by (10). The development of microscopes using the new light-emitting diode (LED) technology as a luminosity source, in substitution to the conventional mercury vapor lamp-based fluorescence microscopes, has made AuO staining a feasible method for, in-field, sputum examination, suitable for low-income settings (reviewed by (10); (11). Higher sensitivity and specificity, comparable to that obtained with the classical AFB staining, have been achieved with LED reading of AuO-stained smears. Moreover, reduced inter-reader variability has been reported with LED reading of AuO-stained smears [11].

7.2.2. Culture of Biological Specimens in New Media and Use of Automated Systems

The culture of mycobacteria followed by species identification by colony morphology and biochemical analysis is still regarded as a gold-standard to be used as a comparison in the evaluation of the performance of newly proposed diagnostic tests [12]. It can achieve high sensitivity, detecting amount as low as 100 bacilli per mL of sample [13], and it is very specific [2]. However, its performance is highly variable among different laboratories, while it requires trained personnel as well as facilities capable of containing the increased risk of airborne spread of bacilli inherent to the procedure [1].

To liquefy respiratory specimens and to avoid contamination of mycobacterial cultures with other bacteria or fungi, a previous decontamination/disaggregation step is performed, which consists in the incubation of samples with sodium hydroxide [14], N-Acetyl-L-Cysteine plus NaOH, or C18-carboxypropylbetaine (C18) [15, 16]. This process improves culture sensitivity, and may have additional positive effects on the sensitivity of AFB smear observation and nucleic acid amplification test (NAAT) performance in the same samples [16].

The solid medium culture method more widely used is the Petroff method, in which digested and decontaminated sputum is centrifuged, neutralized and inoculated in an egg-based medium, Lowenstein-Jensen. Other methods available are the swab method, that uses a sterilized swab to capture relevant material from sputum, followed by decontamination of the material in the scrub and inoculation in a modified egg-based medium (Ogawa modified medium), and the Petroff-Kudoh-Ogawa (PKO) method, that adds the concentration step of Petroff method to the swab method and uses a shorter incubation time for sample decontamination [14]. Time to growth of *M. tuberculosis* cultures in solid medium usually ranges from 2 to 8 weeks [17]. Recently, a new solid medium has been made available, which allows the identification of mycobacterial growth within two weeks, prior to the visual detection of colonies. This is achieved due to the incorporation of indicator dyes to the medium, which signal the presence of mycobacterial metabolites released during growth. On the other hand, the presence of frequently occurring contaminants, instead of mycobacteria, is also signaled by a change in the medium to a different color [18].

Liquid cultures can be more sensitive to detect mycobacteria than cultures in solid media [16; 19-21]. Culture systems using liquid media (modified 7H9, 7H12 or other broth) allow the detection of mycobacterial growth within shorter culture times, typically around 2 weeks, and reduce worker manipulation of bacilli. Initially, semi-automatic liquid culture systems were made available, which used radio-labeled carbon and radiometric detection of this isotope to monitor bacterial growth [13]. These systems have been replaced more recently by fully automated systems that rely on the measurement of changes in gas pressure, carbon dioxide production or oxygen consumption for bacterial growth monitoring, based on the use of fluorescence, colorimetrical or gas-pressure detectors [13, 20, 22]. As the systems that allow automated handling of liquid cultures are expensive, qualitative, non-automated, easy to handle liquid culture systems have been pointed as more realistic and promising tools for low-resource settings [17].

In spite of the availability of fully automated liquid culture procedures, confirmatory cultures in solid media are recommended, as the risk of contamination of liquid cultures is high, especially for non-experienced staffs [1, 17]. The combined use of liquid and solid cultures also increases the detection of bacilli in smear-negative specimens [16]. Small differences have been reported in the performance of commercially available liquid culture systems [13, 20, 21, 23, 24].

Box 1. Commercially Available Nucleic Acid Amplification Tests for Detection of Resistance in *M. tuberculosis* Isolates.

Test	Sequence recognized	Test type	Specimen
Genotype MTBDR*sl*	*gyrA* and *embB* DNA plus16S rRNA of *M. tuberculosis*	semi-quantitative reverse hybridization of PCR product to membrane-bound probes	sputum
Genotype MTBDR*plus*	*rpoB*, *katG* and *inhA* DNA of *M. tuberculosis*	semi-quantitative reverse hybridization of PCR product to membrane-bound probes	sputum
INNO-LIPA Rif TB	*rpoB* DNA of *M. tuberculosis*	semi-quantitative reverse hybridization of PCR product to membrane-bound probes	culture
Xpert MTB/RIF, Cepheid	*rpoB* DNA of *M. tuberculosis*	hemi-nested automated PCR	sputum

PCR: polymerase chain reaction.

Culture methods are also suitable for drug susceptibility testing [18; 25-28] and species identification. M. tuberculosis complex (MTBC) can be distinguished from environmental, non-tuberculous mycobacteria (NTM) based on colony morphology, time of growth, biochemical tests [29], or selective growth inhibition in the presence of ρ-nitro-α-acetylamino-β-hydroxypropiophenone (NAP) or ρ-nitrobenzoic acid (PNB) [18; 22; 30]. It should be observed that available solid and liquid media have been shown to differ in their capacity of supporting the growth of the various mycobacterial species [20; 23]. The identification of mycobacterial species and drug testing, in solid or liquid cultures, can also be performed using NAATs (Box 1).

7.3. MOLECULAR

7.3.1. Nucleic Acid Amplification Tests

Nucleic acid amplification tests (NAATs) rely on the demonstration of MTBC-specific nucleic acid sequences in relevant biological specimens (Box **2**). The methods commercially available have been recently reviewed [31]. The target sequences amplified and detected by most of the currently available assays are depicted below:

- IS*6110* repeated sequence, a mobile element of 1,361 nucleotides present in MTBC [32];

- rDNA or rRNA of the 16S ribosomal subunit of MTBC, as this sequence is an advantageous target for the identification of bacterial species in general [33].

The major limitation for the use of NAATs is the necessity of expensive machines, especially for automated sample processing. Recently, a rapid method of isothermal amplification of DNA has been developed that allows visual detection of the presence of different pathogens in clinical samples without the need of thermocycling machines, and with limited specimen manipulation. The sensitivity of the technique for the detection of mycobacteria has been found to be high for smear-positive samples, but low for smear-negative ones [34, 35].

Box 2. Commercially Available Diagnostic Nucleic Acid Amplification Tests Based on the Recognition of Sequences from the *M. tuberculosis* Complex.

Test	Sequence recognized	Test type	Specimen
Amplified M. tuberculosis Direct Test (MTD, AMTD), Gen-Probe	16S rRNA of *M. tuberculosis* complex	automated transcriptional-mediated amplification	sputum, bronchial specimens, tracheal aspirates
COBAS TaqMan MTB Test	16S rRNA of *M. tuberculosis* complex	automated RT/real-time PCR	respiratory clinical specimens
BDProbeTec ET Direct TB System	IS*6110* DNA of *M. tuberculosis* complex	semi-automated real-time PCR	respiratory and non-pulmonary clinical specimens
Seeplex MTB Nested ACE Detection, Seegene	IS*6110* and MPB64 DNA of *M. tuberculosis* complex	automated nested PCR	sputum, body fluid, bronchial washing, urine, stool, CSF, bone marrow aspiration and tissue (paraffin-embedded), other
Seeplex MTB/BCG ACE Detection, Seegene	RD1 DNA of *M. tuberculosis*	automated nested PCR	sputum, body fluid, bronchial washing, urine, stool, CSF, and bone marrow aspiration
GenoQuick MTB, Hain Lifescience GmbH	?	NASBA and lateral-flow-dipstick hybridization	respiratory and non-pulmonary clinical specimens

PCR: polymerase chain reaction; RT: reverse transcription; CSF: cerebrospinal fluid.

The overall performance of some of the commercially available NAATs has been addressed in systematic review [1] and meta-analysis [3, 36, 37] studies. NAATs have been found to have high specificity, with higher accuracy for respiratory samples [1], but low sensitivity, especially in biological samples where bacilli are rarer (such as cerebrospinal [38] or pleural fluids [39], gastric aspirates [40], biopsies [41], and sputum with low number of bacilli [42]). The sensitivity of NAATs can be comparable to that of conventional smear examination in some of these situations [43]. Some studies have shown good results with extrapulmonary specimens [44, 45], which may be related to the high quality of tested samples [1]. Pulmonary tuberculosis diagnosis in children using NAAT has been reported to achieve high sensitivity and specificity, again with lower performance for smear-negative samples [46]. A recent meta-analysis has shown that both sensitivity and specificity of some commercially available NAATs are highly variable for tuberculous lymphadenitis, a form of tuberculosis that is especially frequent in children and in tuberculosis and HIV co-infected individuals [36]. The reported performance of NAATs for the detection of tuberculous meningitis, another disease form with increased prevalence among pediatric cases, is also low [38]. Unfortunately, these issues limit the usefulness of NAATs for the diagnosis of tuberculosis among infants [47].

The presence of enzymes in respiratory secretions that are capable of inhibiting the amplification reaction accounts for a considerable proportion of false-negative results [3]. This problem can be detected by the inclusion of internal controls, consisting of nucleic acid fragments that are added to each sample and must be co-amplified and detected concomitantly to nucleic acid from mycobacteria in the specimen [48; 49]. On the other hand, carryover of amplycons, polymerase chain reaction (PCR) products from previous or concomitant amplifications is an issue that can lead to false-positive results [3]. Carryover from pre-amplified products can be prevented by the substitution of dUTP for dTTP in the PCR reaction, and digestion of possible carryover prior to new amplification using uracyl-N-glycosilase (UNG) [48; 50]. However, this method does not rule out the possibility of false-positive results, and UNG may be incompletely inactivated in the PCR reaction, resulting in diminished detection of products [51].

Box 3. Commercially Available Nucleic Acid Amplification Tests for Identification of *Mycobacterium* Isolates.

Test	Sequence recognized	Test type	Specimen
AccuProbe *M. tuberculosis* and *M. avium* complexes, *M. intracellulare*, *M. avium* complex, *M. kansasii*, *M. gordonae*; Gen-Probe	mycobacterium 16S rDNA	automated nested PCR	culture
COBAS Amplicor *M. avium*, *M. intracellulare* Test; Roche Diagnostics	mycobacterium 16S rRNA	automated RT/real-time PCR	respiratory clinical specimens
Seeplex MTBC/NTM ACE Detection, Seegene	mycobacterium IS*6110* and MPB64 DNA	dual-priming oligonucleotide multiplex PCR	culture
Genotype MTBC, Hain Lifescience GmbH	23S rDNA, *gyrB* and RD1 DNA of MTBC	semi-quantitative reverse hybridization of PCR product to membrane-bound probes	culture
Genotype *Mycobacterium* CM/AS, Hain Lifescience GmbH	mycobacterium 23S rDNA	semi-quantitative reverse hybridization of PCR product to membrane-bound probes	culture
INNO-LiPA Mycobacteria v2, Innogenetics	16S-23S rDNA spacer region of mycobacteria	semi-quantitative reverse hybridization of PCR product to membrane-bound probes	culture

PCR: polymerase chain reaction; RT: reverse transcription.

The identification of *Mycobacterium* species can also be performed with the help of NAATs (Box **3**). The discrimination of mycobacterial species causing disease is important, as NTM can cause tuberculous-like disease and may be resistant to anti-tuberculosis drugs [52]. NAATs sensitivity and specificity for the identification of *Mycobacterium* species has been found to be high for isolates of both MTBC [53-55] and *M. avium* complex [53, 55], as well as for other mycobacteria [56-59].

Drug-resistant *M. tuberculosis* strains can also be demonstrated in clinical isolates with these methods. High sensitivity and specificity have been reported for the detection of mutations in the *rpoB* gene [60; 61], as well as for *katG* and *inhA* [60], *gyrA* and *rrs* [62], but low sensitivity has been found for *embB* [62]. Please, again, refer to Box **1**, above, for the lists of available tests that use NAAT to detect resistant isolates.

7.3.2. Phage-Based Detection of Mycobacteria in Short Term Cultures of Clinical Specimens

Phages are viruses that replicate inside bacteria (lysogenic phase) thereby lysing the bacterial host (lytic phase). When bacteria are cultured in plates with solid medium in the presence of phages that recognize them, bacterial lysis by these viruses can be observed as cleared spots or disappearance of the whole bacterial lawn. Some mycobacteriophages have been identified which can infect only a narrow range of mycobacterial species, and therefore have been explored for molecular diagnostic tests [63].

As members of the MTBC have a slow growth, "helper" cells, consisting of fast-growing *M. smegmatis*, are used to facilitate in visualize the occurrence of phage infection that signals the presence of viable mycobacteria originally in the clinical specimen. Following decontamination and concentration, clinical specimens are submitted to overnight culture in liquid media, and then exposed to mycobateriophages for a few minutes to allow infection of viable bacilli. After this, samples are promptly incubated with a virucidal solution to inactivate those phages that remain extracellular. "Helper" cells are added to the culture, and the sample is plated in melted agar, and then incubated overnight. The continuous lawn of *M. smegmatis* will present a number of lytic plates (above any given threshold) if viable phages were present in the initial sample that survived the virucidal solution, since they had found viable mycobacteria to host them [64; 65]. As the method allows the identification of viable bacilli, the phage assays have also been adapted to detect drug-susceptibility strains using short-term cultures [66; 67].

The sensitivity and positive predictive value of phage tests has been found to be highly variable [68]. Diminished sensitivity has been found for smear-negative specimens [69; 70]. Other factors that contribute to a lower sensitivity are the contamination of agar plates, which can be frequent and may impair test reading, and the sample transport conditions, which may reduce bacterial viability [71]. Contamination can be reduced with the use of antibiotic supplementation [72]. Regarding the drug susceptibility testing, *M. tuberculosis* isolates with low-level susceptibility may also be more difficult to detect [73]. However, the test has been found to be rapid and of low cost, and useful for screening in low-income settings [73-75].

7.4. IMMUNOLOGICAL

7.4.1. Detection of Mycobacterium Antigens or Anti-Mycobacterium Antibodies

The identification of (i) soluble, excreted mycobacterial antigens in urine samples [76] or specimen filtrates [77, 78], or (ii) serum antibodies against mycobacterial products from the immunoglobulins (Ig)G, IgM, or IgA antibody classes [79], has provided the basis for many rapid diagnostic tests for tuberculosis. These tests are generally based on antibody recognition of target molecules in immunochromatography or immunoenzymatic assays (Box **4**).

Whole mycobacteria of the MTBC, present in dissolved/filtrated specimens, such as sputum, urine, pus, biopsies, as well as bronchial, lymph node, pleural or gastric aspirates, can be detected directly using polyclonal antibodies against mycobacterial compounds [78]. On the other hand, antibodies against specific components can be used in immunodiagnostic assays to demonstrate the presence of bacilli. One example is the MPB-64 protein of MTBC [77, 80]. The antigen MPB-64 is a 24-kDa protein abundantly secreted by MTBC, with well characterized B-cell epitopes [81], and a member of a small family of proteins that are highly conserved among these bacteria, however, with no homology with other known proteins [82]. The detection of this antigen is possible in cultures performed with liquid or solid media. This method has been found to have high sensitivity and specificity, but cultures with low numbers of bacilli can yield false-negative results, and some strains lacking the expression of MPB-64 due to mutations in this gene have been reported [77].

The detection of mycobacterial lipoarabinomannan (LAM) has also been explored in immunodiagnostic tests using urine samples. LAM is an important component of the *M. tuberculosis* cell wall, consisting of multi-glycosilated extensions of phosphatidyl-inositol manosides, anchored in the plasma membrane by phosphatidylinositol moieties [83]. LAM is released inside *Mycobacterium*-containing phagosomes [83] and reaches the blood of tuberculosis patients with active disease, being detectable in urine samples from tuberculosis patients without modifications [84]. LAM antigen concentration in urine has been strongly correlated with the microscopic density of mycobacteria in the sputum of pulmonary tuberculosis patients [85], but the technique has shown low sensitivity for disease detection [86]. LAM detection in urine has also been evaluated in populations with high HIV prevalence, in which it has achieved low sensitivity [84; 87], and negative predictive value [84]. This is especially telling when comparing smear- and culture-positive patients with smear- and culture-negative treated subjects or individuals with pulmonary disease other than tuberculosis [84, 87]. Among tuberculosis and HIV co-infected patients, detectable LAM has been strongly associated with low CD4 T cell counts and advanced clinical stage, and possibly also with immune reconstitution inflammatory syndrome [88].

Several immunological tests have been developed to detect serum antibodies against mycobacterial compounds, and their efficacy has been tested both alone and in combination with each other [79, 89-91]. Most of the tests detect antibodies that recognize mycobacterial proteins, such as A60 [91-94], 38-kDa [79, 91], or other [12, 79], but some of them detect antibodies against *M. tuberculosis* glycolipids, such as LAM [90, 95], or other [90, 96]. The humoral immune response is believed to correlate with disease progression from the latent to the active form [91], nonetheless, the performance of available tests in recognizing this transition has not been reported so far. In general, the literature evaluating serological tests shows poor sensitivity [1, 97, 98] as well as low positive and negative predictive value [76, 93, 94], and so the search for better markers of tuberculosis disease continues.

The accuracy of serological tests may be influenced by disease stage, exposure to NTM, atypical mycobacteria, Bacille Calmette-Guerin (BCG) vaccination and HIV infection [1]. There is also high individual variability among different tuberculosis patients in the profile of antibody reactivity [99]. Past tuberculosis treatment has been associated with increased proportion of false-positive results [12], limiting the utility of these tests in high-disease burden settings. Reported performance of immunoassays for smear-negative tuberculosis cases has been lower than that obtained for smear-positive cases in several studies [76, 96], which is of concern as new tests would ideally help in the diagnosis of smear-negative patients. In children with pulmonary tuberculosis, the available tests seem to yield results comparable to those found in adults [93]. However, for children with extrapulmonary tuberculosis, antibody detection of some antigens may be lower [76]. The overall performance of commercially available serological tests for the diagnosis of pulmonary [97] and extrapulmonary [98] antigens of *M. tuberculosis* has been systematically reviewed and will not be the main focus of the present chapter.

Of note, the detection of biomarkers of tuberculosis disease has also been explored in non-immune blood assays. Thus, the jellification of blood samples upon exposure to glutaraldehyde (Box **4**) occurs faster in blood from humans and cattle with tuberculosis in comparison to blood from normal individuals [100, 101]. It has been hypothesized that high levels of fibrinogen and gammaglobulins, associated with decreased fibrinolysis and accentuated platelet aggregation, could account for this phenomenon [101]. Some studies of in-house tests have been carried out to explore the performance of this methodology; in these studies, both sensitivity and specificity were found to be above 80% [100-102]. However, the literature lacks studies regarding the performance of such tests in children, extrapulmonary disease patients or HIV-infected subjects.

Box 4. Commercially Available Tests Based on the Recognition of Mycobacterial Antigens or of Serum Antibodies Against Mycobacterium Components.

Test	Antigen recognized	Specimen
Anda-TB GA Test, Anda Biologicals	Elevated gammaglobulin and fibrinogen (non-mycobacterial)	blood
Clearview TB ELISA, Clearview	LAM	urine
Capilia TB (ICT), Find Diagnostics/Tauns Co.	MPB64 of *M. tuberculosis* complex	cultures in liquid/solid media
Anda-TB (ELISA), Anda Biologicals	anti-mycobacterial A60 IgM, IgA, IgG or IgM/IgG	serum, saliva, sputum, CSF, other fluids
PATHOZYME-TB complex plus (ELISA), Omega Diagnostics	anti-*M. tuberculosis* 38-kDa and 16-kDa IgG	serum
PATHOZYME-MYCO (ELISA), Omega Diagnostics	anti-LAM plus anti-*M. tuberculosis* 38-kDa IgM, IgA or IgG	serum
ActiveTb*Detect* ELISA, InBios International	anti-mycobacterium Mtb8, Mtb81, Mtb48, MPT32, 38-kDa IgM or IgG and 2 other	serum
IBL *M.tuberculosis* ELISA, IBL-Hamburg GmbH	anti-mycobacterial 18-kDa, 36-kDa and 40-kDa IgM, IgA or IgG	serum, plasma
Determiner TBGL antibody, Kyowa Medex	Ig against tuberculous glycolipids	serum
MycoDot (ICT), Mosmann Associates	Anti-LAM Ig	whole-blood, serum or plasma

ELISA: enzyme-linked immunosorbent assay; ICT: immunochromatography; LAM: lipoarabinomannan; CSF: cerebrospinal fluid.

7.4.2. Detection of Specific T Cells-Secreting Cytokines

M. tuberculosis infection elicits the immune response of the host, resulting in the expansion of *M. tuberculosis*-specific T cells that secrete a myriad of cytokines in the presence of mycobacterial antigens. One of the cytokines that is highly produced by infected or diseased individuals in response to *in vitro* mycobacterial challenge is interferon-gamma (IFN-γ). Both the frequency of *M. tuberculosis*-specific IFN-γ-secreting T cells and the levels of IFN-γ in whole-blood cultures performed in the presence of specific *M. tuberculosis* antigens are increased in those individuals with active or latent tuberculosis disease in comparison with healthy subjects [103, 104], and this has been used as the rationale for the development of diagnostic assays for the assessment of *M. tuberculosis* infection in substitution to the TST [105, 106]. Those tests are broadly known as IGRAs, the initials for Interferon-Gamma Release Assay.

Of particular interest for diagnosis is the assessment of the IFN-γ response to the specific mycobacterial antigens encoded by the region of difference (RD)-1 of MTBC, as this sequence, although present in *M. bovis*, is absent in the BCG vaccine strains, or in the majority of NTM. This allows the discrimination between the immune response to infecting MTBC and the specific response to previous BCG vaccination, or elicited by encounter with NTM (which have both been shown to induce immunity that may interfere with the read out of the gold-standard test for latent disease, the TST or Mantoux test). Among the specific *M. tuberculosis* antigens commonly used in commercially available diagnostic tests based on this approach are the extensively studied early secretory antigenic target (ESAT)-6 and culture filtrate protein (CFP)-10 proteins. Lalvani and Pareek (2009) [107] performed a comprehensive review on this subject.

Due to the lack of a gold-standard to define the true specificity and sensitivity of latent tuberculosis assessment, the degree of agreement between IGRA and TST results, their performance in correlating with the level of exposure to index cases of tuberculosis, and in identifying subjects with active disease (as a surrogate of infected individuals) has been assessed [107]. Each of these approaches has its drawbacks, as

TST positivity is not always associated with latent infection, the correlation with level of exposure does not allow the determination of sensitivity or specificity, and individuals with active disease, especially immunecompromised patients, can have diminished production of IFN-γ, mostly leading to indeterminate results.

IGRA tests based on either ELISpot or ELISA cytokine detection have both shown to correlate well with the level of patient exposure to index cases of tuberculosis, and not to be influenced by BCG vaccination status, as expected. The specificity of IGRAs in determining latent tuberculosis has been shown to be higher than the specificity of TST, which is consistent with the fact that these tests are not influenced by the immune response to previous vaccination. IGRA tests based on ELISA cytokine detection in the supernatant have presented more variable levels of agreement with TST. The sensitivity of ELISpot-based platform has been shown to be higher than the sensitivity of ELISA-based platform among immunecompromised individuals, particularly among HIV-positive, malnourished patients, and children under 3-years old, but ELISpot assays have also been found to be more influenced by previous tuberculosis disease [107].

7.4.2.1. Assays Based on Interferon-Gamma Detection in the Supernatants by ELISA

Previously, these assays have been developed for the determination of tuberculosis infection in cattle, and later in humans [105, 106]. The most recent commercially available form of the test for humans, the QuantiFERON®-TB Gold In-Tube (QFT-GIT) has an Australian patent under the Cellestis Inc., and compares the IFN-γ release in the supernates of whole-blood cultures of the same individual, in three experimental conditions: nil tube (absence of stimulus), a mitogen (upon phytohemagglutinin stimulation), or upon stimulation with three *M. tuberculosis* RD-1 antigens (CFP-10, ESAT-6 and TB7.7). Lately, IFN-γ is detected in the supernatant by an ordinary ELISA.

Positivity to QFT-GIT has been found to have better correlation with longer exposure to index case of tuberculosis than TST. The agreement between both tests has been found to be associated with higher sputum-smear bacillary load of the index case [108]. Both sensitivity and specificity of QFT-GIT have been shown to be higher than those of TST for the detection of active tuberculosis [109]. On the other hand, given a TST cut-off of 10 mm, the rate of progression to tuberculosis disease among untreated QFT-GIT positive subjects was found to be equivalent to the rate of progression to disease among untreated TST-positive subjects [110].

In a study performed in Germany, QFT-GIT positivity in the absence of TST positivity was associated with aging, independently of BCG vaccination status or the risk factors for latent tuberculosis, such as being foreign-born or health-care worker [111]. That same scenario was also found to be associated with absence of lung scar by chest X-ray, as well as with non-cavitary disease among contacts of an index case of tuberculosis in Brazil [108]. In another study, QFT-GIT positive but TST-negative, results have been associated with severe underlying diseases, immunesuppressive treatment and past tuberculosis [112]. There is no agreement as to whether chemoprophylaxis should be recommended in such cases.

In children, low to moderate agreement between TST and QFT-GIT results has been observed among non-BCG vaccinated individuals, considering TST higher than 15 mm as the regular cut-off [113, 114]. QFT-GIT positivity in children has been more associated with recent exposure to a known case of tuberculosis [114].

7.4.2.2. Assays Quantifying the Frequency of Interferon-Gamma Producing Cells by ELISpot

ELISpot detection of IFN-γ-releasing T cells is the rational basis of two presently commercially available tests for latent tuberculosis diagnosis: The T-SPOT®.*TB* under a British patent from Oxford based Immunotec, and the ELISpot^PRO® / ELISpot^PLUS® under a Swedish, Mabtech, patent. In these tests, the frequency of IFN-γ released by T cells, (revealed as fingerprints by means of spots in the subjacent polyvinyl-difluoride membrane), is compared among peripheral blood mononuclear cell cultures performed either in the absence of antigen, the presence of a mitogen (phytohemagglutinin) or in the presence of a number of peptide pools corresponding to overlapping aminoacid sequences from either specific *M. tuberculosis* ESAT-6 or CFP-10 proteins.

The ELISpot[PLUS®] assay has been shown to be as sensitive as the TST for latent tuberculosis detection [115]. Higher concordance has been found between T-SPOT®.*TB* and QFT-GIT results than between T-SPOT®.*TB* and TST [116, 117].

Similarly to what has been found for QFT-GIT (see section 7.4.2.1.), the discordance between T-SPOT®.*TB* and TST results cannot be explained only by previous BCG vaccination, and there is no consensus as to whether individuals with a positive T-SPOT®.*TB* result, but negative TST would be eligible for chemoprophylaxis to treat latent tuberculosis [118]. T-SPOT®.*TB* positivity in the absence of TST-positive results has been associated with intravenous drug use [119]. Individuals with indeterminate results for QFT-GIT can be correctly diagnosed with tuberculosis after being tested with T-SPOT®.*TB*. Indeterminate results obtained with this technique have been associated with aging and decreased serum protein and albumin, two parameters associated with hyponutrition [120].

Among children in contact with index cases of tuberculosis, test positivity has been found to be higher for T-SPOT®.*TB* than for TST, in agreement with a higher specificity of latent detection for T-SPOT®.*TB*. On the other hand, the rate of progression to active tuberculosis disease was similar among T-SPOT®.*TB*- and TST-positive individuals [121]. High diagnostic sensitivity and specificity has been found for detection of tuberculous meningitis among HIV-negative children, using either cerebrospinal fluid or blood cultures [122]. A typical ELISpot result can be found in the append section.

7.5. PERSPECTIVES IN THE DIAGNOSIS OF ACTIVE AND LATENT TUBERCULOSIS IN CHILDREN

A flowchart was assembled to illustrate a possible decision tree for the application of diagnostic tests in different contexts of tuberculosis management (Fig. **1**).

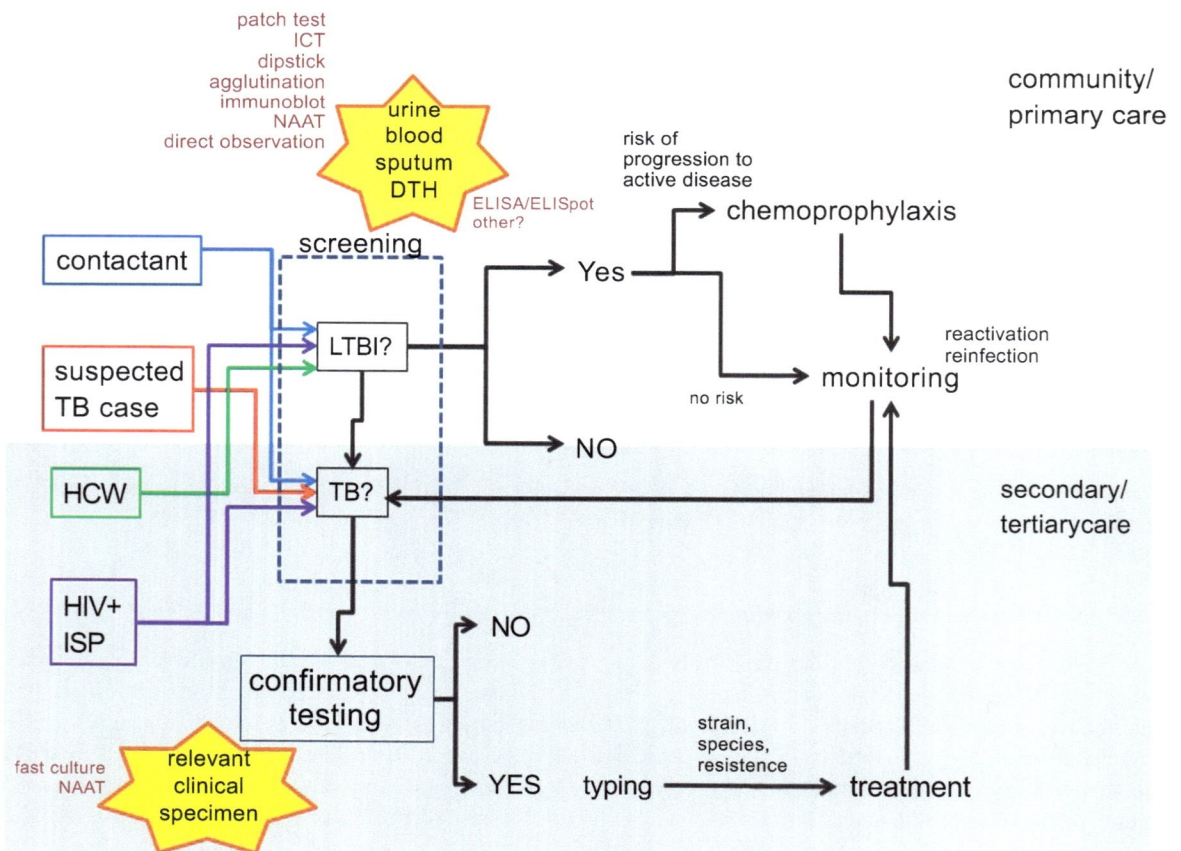

Fig. (1). Flowchart for the application of new diagnostic measures in different contexts of tuberculosis management.

ELISA, enzyme-linked immunosorbent assay; ELISpot, enzyme-linked immunospot assay; ICT, immunochromatography; NAAT, nucleic acid amplification test; DTH, delayed-type hypersensitivity; TB, tuberculosis; LTBI, latent tuberculosis infection; HCW, health-care worker; HIV+, human immunodeficiency virus-infected patient; ISP, immunesuppressed patient.

Suspected disease cases and contactants, health-care workers, as well as immunesuppressed individuals (including HIV-positive subjects) would be ideally screened for tuberculosis disease or latent infection. This would be done by using low complexity, rapid diagnostic, assays that proved to have high negative predictive value as well as high sensitivity. It should also follow that it has reproducibility in the field for the multiplicity of disease forms. Priority would be given for those tests that would be less invasive, and, in the case of latent tuberculosis, that could help in the establishment of the risk of progression to active disease. Confirmatory tests following a positive result in this initial screening should have a high positive predictive value. They would, ideally, not require new sample collection, concomitantly allowing the assessment of mycobacterial species and drug resistance, while even typing for strains of clinical importance. These tests should give a rapid response for treatment decision-making, thereby contributing to diminish the contagiousness of pulmonary cases and allowing for the rational implementation of chemoprophylaxis schemes in latently infected individuals.

In addition to the World Health Organization published recommendations [123], in children only IGRAs have been recommended as alternative confirmatory tests for active tuberculosis, (in substitution to TST), as well as potentially better diagnostic tests for latent infection, (especially among BCG-vaccinated children). Nonetheless, negative results should not necessarily be interpreted as an absence of infection; IGRA results are also not indicative of progression to disease [124].

Achieving a more efficient and accurate diagnosis of tuberculosis is an essential arm to its control. The improvement in the detection rates will reduce the time to management of the disease and will, therefore, impact the duration of infectiousness and disease progression; furthermore, it will limit the severity, contributing to a decrease in mortality and transmission rates [17, 125].

7.6. CONCLUDING REMARKS

Here, the laboratory methods presented exemplify some of the strategies that have been achieved by the market as potential improvements for the diagnosis of tuberculosis. The implementation of each of these methods in the routine management of the disease has been hampered by one or more of the following:

- Scarcity of validation studies to establish their accuracy and reproducibility in field work.

- Use of instruments of elevated complexity.

- High cost and training required for their implementation.

- Variable performance observed in studies conducted in different settings.

Given the complexity of the disease, it is likely that a combination of strategies will need to be employed to circumvent those bottlenecks, and such diagnostic flowcharts, depicted early, should be proposed and tested for cost-effectiveness in the in-field settings.

REFERENCES

[1]   Dinnes J, Deeks J, Kunst H, *et al.* A systematic review of rapid diagnostic tests for the detection of tuberculosis infection. Health Technol Assess 2007; 11(3): 1-196.

[2]   Davies PD, Pai M. The diagnosis and misdiagnosis of tuberculosis (state of the art series - No. 1). Int J Tuberc Lung Dis 2008; 12(11): 1226-34.

[3]   Greco S, Girardi E, Navarra A, Saltini C. Current evidence on diagnostic accuracy of commercially based nucleic acid amplification tests for the diagnosis of pulmonary tuberculosis. Thorax 2006; 61(9): 783-90.

[4]   Siddiqi K, Lambert ML, Walley J. Clinical diagnosis of smear-negative pulmonary tuberculosis in low-income countries: the current evidence. Lancet Infect Dis 2003; 3(5): 288-96.

[5]   Steingart KR, Henry M, Ng V, *et al.* Fluorescence versus conventional sputum smear microscopy for tuberculosis: a systematic review. Lancet Infect Dis 2006; 6: 570-81.

[6]   Steingart KR, Ng V, Henry M, *et al.* Sputum processing methods to improve the sensitivity of smear microscopy for tuberculosis: a systematic review. Lancet Infect Dis 2006; 6(10): 664-74.

[7]   Centers for Disease Control and Prevention. Controlling Tuberculosis in the United States: Recommendations from the American Thoracic Society, CDC, and the Infectious Diseases Society of America. MMWR; 2005. Report No. 54.

[8]   Sharma RK, Rajput KP, Kothari ND, Nerurkar V, Malvankar SS. Pilot evaluation of commercial liquid culture method for isolation of mycobacteria in resource-poor settings. Indian J Med Microbiol 2009; 27(4): 374-5.

[9]   Brent AJ, Anderson ST, Kampmann B. Childhood tuberculosis: Out of sight, out of mind? Trans R Soc Trop Med Hyg 2008; 102(3): 217-8.

[10]   Hanscheid T. The future looks bright: Low-cost fluorescent microscopes for detection of *Mycobacterium tuberculosis* and coccidiae. Trans R Soc Trop Med Hyg 2008; 102(6): 520-1.

[11]   Marais BJ, Brittle W, Painczyk K, *et al.* Use of light-emitting diode fluorescence microscopy to detect acid-fast bacilli in sputum. Clin Infect Dis 2008; 47: 203-7.

[12]   Al Zahrani K, Al Jahdali H, Poirier L, Rene P, Gennaro ML, Menzies D. Accuracy and utility of commercially available amplification and serologic tests for the diagnosis of minimal pulmonary tuberculosis. Am J Respir Crit Care Med 2000; 162(4): 1323-8.

[13]   Palomino JC. Nonconventional and new methods in the diagnosis of tuberculosis: feasibility and applicability in the field. Eur Respir J 2005; 26(2): 339-50.

[14]   Salem JI, Carvalho CM, Ogusko MM, Maia R, Ruffino-Netto A. Alternative method for isolating Mycobacteria from sputum. Acta Amazonica 2007; 37(3): 419-24.

[15]   Scott CP, Dos Anjos Filho L, De Queiroz Mello *et al.* Comparison of C(18)-carboxypropylbetaine and standard N-acetyl-L-cysteine-NaOH processing of respiratory specimens for increasing tuberculosis smear sensitivity in Brazil. J Clin Microbiol 2002; 40(9): 3219-22.

[16]   Padilla E, Manterola JM, Gonzalez V, *et al.* Comparison of the sodium hydroxide specimen processing method with the C18-carboxypropylbetaine specimen processing method using independent specimens with auramine smear, the MB/BacT liquid culture system, and the COBAS AMPLICOR MTB test. J Clin Microbiol 2005; 43(12): 6091-7.

[17]   Perkins MD, Cunningham J. Facing the crisis: improving the diagnosis of tuberculosis in the HIV era. J Infect Dis 2007; 196(1): 15-27.

[18]   Baylan O, Kisa O, Albay A, Doganci L. Evaluation of a new automated, rapid, colorimetric culture system using solid medium for laboratory diagnosis of tuberculosis and determination of anti-tuberculosis drug susceptibility. Int J Tuberc Lung Dis 2004; 8(6): 772-7.

[19]   Tholcken CA, Huang S, Woods GL. Evaluation of the ESP Culture System II for recovery of mycobacteria from blood specimens collected in isolator tubes. J Clin Microbiol 1997; 35(10): 2681-2.

[20]   Woods GL, Fish G, Plaunt M, Murphy T. Clinical evaluation of DIFCO ESP culture system II for growth and detection of mycobacteria. J Clin Microbiol 1997; 35(1): 121-4.

[21]   Somoskovi A, Magyar P. Comparison of the mycobacteria growth indicator tube with MB redox, Lowenstein-Jensen, and Middlebrook 7H11 media for recovery of mycobacteria in clinical specimens. J Clin Microbiol 1999; 37(5): 1366-9.

[22]   Gross WM, Hawkins JE. Radiometric selective inhibition tests for differentiation of *Mycobacterium tuberculosis*, *Mycobacterium bovis*, and other mycobacteria. J Clin Microbiol 1985; 21(4): 565-8.

[23]   Piersimoni C, Scarparo C, Callegaro A, *et al.* Comparison of MB/Bact alert 3D system with radiometric BACTEC system and Lowenstein-Jensen medium for recovery and identification of mycobacteria from clinical specimens: a multicenter study. J Clin Microbiol 2001; 39(2): 651-7.

[24]   Sorlozano A, Soria I, Roman J, *et al.* Comparative evaluation of three culture methods for the isolation of mycobacteria from clinical samples. J Microbiol Biotechnol 2009; 19(10): 1259-64.

[25]   Adjers-Koskela K, Katila ML. Susceptibility testing with the manual mycobacteria growth indicator tube (MGIT) and the MGIT 960 system provides rapid and reliable verification of multidrug-resistant tuberculosis. J Clin Microbiol 2003; 41(3): 1235-8.

[26]   Ani AE, Daylop YB, Agbaji O, Idoko J. Drug susceptibility test of *Mycobacterium tuberculosis* by nitrate reductase assay. J Infect Dev Ctries 2009; 3(1): 16-9.

[27]   Ogwang S, Asiimwe BB, Traore H, *et al.* Comparison of rapid tests for detection of rifampicin-resistant *Mycobacterium tuberculosis* in Kampala, Uganda. BMC Infect Dis 2009; 9: 139-40.

[28]   Verma JS, Rawat D, Hasan A, *et al.* The use of E-test for the drug susceptibility testing of *Mycobacterium tuberculosis* - a solution or an illusion? Indian J Med Microbiol 2010; 28(1): 30-3.

[29]   Konno K. New chemical method to differentiate human-type tubercle bacilli from other mycobacteria. Science 1956; 124(3229): 985-6.

[30]   Giampaglia CM, Martins MC, Chimara E, Oliveira RS, de Oliveira Vieira GB, Marsico AG, *et al.* Differentiation of *Mycobacterium tuberculosis* from other mycobacteria with rho-nitrobenzoic acid using MGIT960. Int J Tuberc Lung Dis 2007; 11(7): 803-7.

[31]   Neonakis IK, Gitti Z, Krambovitis E, Spandidos DA. Molecular diagnostic tools in mycobacteriology. J Microbiol Methods 2008; 75(1): 1-11.

[32]   Thierry D, Cave MD, Eisenach KD, *et al.* IS6110,an IS-like element of *Mycobacterium tuberculosis* complex. Nucleic Acids Res 1990; 18(1): 188-9.

[33]   Huyghe A, Francois P, Schrenzel J. Characterization of microbial pathogens by DNA microarrays. Infect Genet Evol 2009; 9(5): 987-95.

[34]   Boehme CC, Nabeta P, Henostroza G, *et al.* Operational feasibility of using loop-mediated isothermal amplification for diagnosis of pulmonary tuberculosis in microscopy centers of developing countries. J Clin Microbiol 2007; 45(6): 1936-40.

[35]   Cho S. Current issues on molecular and immunological diagnosis of tuberculosis. Yonsei Med J 2007; 48(3): 347-59.

[36]   Daley P, Thomas S, Pai M. Nucleic acid amplification tests for the diagnosis of tuberculous lymphadenitis: A systematic review. Int J Tuberc Lung Dis 2007; 11(11): 1166-76.

[37]   Ling DI, Flores LL, Riley LW, Pai M. Commercial nucleic-acid amplification tests for diagnosis of pulmonary tuberculosis in respiratory specimens: Meta-analysis and meta-regression. PLoS One 2008; 3(2): 1536-7.

[38]   Thwaites GE, Caws M, Chau TT, *et al.* Comparison of conventional bacteriology with nucleic acid amplification (amplified *Mycobacterium* direct test) for diagnosis of tuberculous meningitis before and after inception of antituberculosis chemotherapy. J Clin Microbiol 2004; 42(3): 996-1002.

[39]   Moon JW, Chang YS, Kim SK, *et al.* The clinical utility of polymerase chain reaction for the diagnosis of pleural tuberculosis. Clin Infect Dis 2005; 41(5): 660-6.

[40]   Mitarai S, Tanoue S, Sugita C, *et al.* Potential use of Amplicor PCR kit in diagnosing pulmonary tuberculosis from gastric aspirate. J Microbiol Methods 2001; 47(3): 339-44.

[41]   Ruiz-Manzano J, Manterola JM, Gamboa F, *et al.* Detection of *Mycobacterium tuberculosis* in paraffin-embedded pleural biopsy specimens by commercial ribosomal RNA and DNA amplification kits. Chest 2000; 118(3): 648-55.

[42]   Noordhoek GT, Mulder S, Wallace P, Van Loon AM. Multicentre quality control study for detection of *Mycobacterium tuberculosis* in clinical samples by nucleic amplification methods. Clin Microbiol Infect 2004; 10(4): 295-301.

[43]   Bayram A, Celiksoz C, Karsligil T, Balci I. Automatized PCR evaluation of *Mycobacterium tuberculosis* complex in respiratory and nonrespiratory specimens. FEMS Immunol Med Microbiol 2006; 46(1): 48-52.

[44]   Ehlers S, Ignatius R, Regnath T, Hahn H. Diagnosis of extrapulmonary tuberculosis by gen-probe amplified *Mycobacterium tuberculosis* direct test. J Clin Microbiol 1996; 34(9): 2275-9.

[45]   Pfyffer GE, Kissling P, Jahn EM, Welscher HM, Salfinger M, Weber R. Diagnostic performance of amplified *Mycobacterium tuberculosis* direct test with cerebrospinal fluid, other nonrespiratory, and respiratory specimens. J Clin Microbiol 1996; 34(4): 834-41.

[46]   Zaki ME, bou-El Hassan S. Clinical evaluation of Gen-Probe's amplified *Mycobacterium tuberculosis* direct test for rapid diagnosis of *Mycobacterium tuberculosis* in Egyptian children at risk for infection. Arch Pathol Lab Med 2008; 132(2): 244-7.

[47]   Cho SN, Brennan PJ. Tuberculosis: Diagnostics. Tuberculosis 2007; 87(1): 14-7.

[48]   Eing BR, Becker A, Sohns A, Ringelmann R. Comparison of Roche Cobas Amplicor *Mycobacterium tuberculosis* assay with in-house PCR and culture for detection of *M. tuberculosis*. J Clin Microbiol 1998; 36(7): 2023-9.

[49]   Rajalahti I, Vuorinen P, Nieminen MM, Miettinen A. Detection of *Mycobacterium tuberculosis* complex in sputum specimens by the automated Roche Cobas Amplicor *Mycobacterium tuberculosis* Test. J Clin Microbiol 1998; 36(4): 975-8.

[50]   Ritzler M, Perschil I, Altwegg M. Influence of residual uracil-DNA glycosylase activity on the electrophoretic migration of dUTP-containing PCR products. J Microbiol Methods 1999; 35(1): 73-6.

[51]   Noordhoek GT, van Embden JD, Kolk AH. Reliability of nucleic acid amplification for detection of *Mycobacterium tuberculosis*: an international collaborative quality control study among 30 laboratories. J Clin Microbiol 1996; 34(10): 2522-5.

[52]   Andrejak C, Lescure FX, Douadi Y, *et al.* Non-tuberculous mycobacteria pulmonary infection: Management and follow-up of 31 infected patients. J Infect 2007; 55(1): 34-40.

[53]   Ninet B, Rohner P, Metral C, Auckenthaler R. Assessment of use of the COBAS AMPLICOR system with BACTEC 12B cultures for rapid detection of frequently identified mycobacteria. J Clin Microbiol 1999; 37(3): 782-4.

[54]   Bergmann JS, Keating WE, Woods GL. Clinical evaluation of the BDProbeTec ET system for rapid detection of *Mycobacterium tuberculosis*. J Clin Microbiol 2000; 38(2): 863-5.

[55]   Katila ML, Katila P, Erkinjuntti-Pekkanen R. Accelerated detection and identification of mycobacteria with MGIT 960 and COBAS AMPLICOR systems. J Clin Microbiol 2000; 38(3): 960-4.

[56]   Scarparo C, Piccoli P, Rigon A, Ruggiero G, Nista D, Piersimoni C. Direct identification of mycobacteria from MB/BacT alert 3D bottles: comparative evaluation of two commercial probe assays. J Clin Microbiol 2001; 39(9): 3222-7.

[57]   Makinen J, Marjamaki M, Marttila H, Soini H. Evaluation of a novel strip test, GenoType *Mycobacterium* CM/AS, for species identification of mycobacterial cultures. Clin Microbiol Infect 2006; 12(5): 481-3.

[58]   Richter E, Weizenegger M, Fahr AM, Rusch-Gerdes S. Usefulness of the GenoType MTBC assay for differentiating species of the *Mycobacterium tuberculosis* complex in cultures obtained from clinical specimens. J Clin Microbiol 2004; 42(9): 4303-6.

[59]   Gitti Z, Neonakis I, Fanti G, Kontos F, Maraki S, Tselentis Y. Use of the GenoType *Mycobacterium* CM and AS assays to analyze 76 nontuberculous mycobacterial isolates from Greece. J Clin Microbiol 2006; 44(6): 2244-6.

[60]   Hillemann D, Rusch-Gerdes S, Richter E. Evaluation of the GenoType MTBDRplus assay for rifampin and isoniazid susceptibility testing of *Mycobacterium tuberculosis* strains and clinical specimens. J Clin Microbiol 2007; 45(8): 2635-40.

[61]   Hauck Y, Fabre M, Vergnaud G, Soler C, Pourcel C. Comparison of two commercial assays for the characterization of rpoB mutations in *Mycobacterium tuberculosis* and description of new mutations conferring weak resistance to rifampicin. J Antimicrob Chemother 2009; 64(2): 259-62.

[62]   Hillemann D, Rusch-Gerdes S, Richter E. Feasibility of the GenoType MTBDRsl assay for fluoroquinolone, amikacin, capreomycin, and ethambutol resistance testing of *Mycobacterium tuberculosis* strains and clinical specimens. J Clin Microbiol 2009; 47(6): 1767-72.

[63]   McNerney R. TB: The Return of The Phage: A review of fifty years of mycobacteriophage research. Int J Tuberc Lung Dis 1999; 3(3): 179-84.

[64]   Albay A, Kisa O, Baylan O, Doganci L. The evaluation of FASTPlaqueTB test for the rapid diagnosis of tuberculosis. Diagn Microbiol Infect Dis 2003; 46(3): 211-5.

[65]   Kiraz N, Et L, Akgun Y, Kasifoglu N, Kiremitci A. Rapid detection of *Mycobacterium tuberculosis* from sputum specimens using the FASTPlaqueTB test. Int J Tuberc Lung Dis 2007; 11(8): 904-8.

[66]   Krishnamurthy A, Rodrigues C, Mehta AP. Rapid detection of rifampicin resistance in *M. tuberculosis* by phage assay. Indian J Med Microbiol 2002; 20(4): 211-4.

[67]   Albert H, Trollip AP, Seaman T, *et al.* Evaluation of a rapid screening test for rifampicin resistance in re-treatment tuberculosis patients in the eastern cape. S Afr Med J 2007; 97(9): 858-63.

[68]   Kalantri S, Pai M, Pascopella L, Riley L, Reingold A. Bacteriophage-based tests for the detection of *Mycobacterium tuberculosis* in clinical specimens: a systematic review and meta-analysis. BMC Infect Dis 2005; 5(1): 59-60.

[69]   Alcaide F, Gali N, Dominguez J, *et al.* Usefulness of a new mycobacteriophage-based technique for rapid diagnosis of pulmonary tuberculosis. J Clin Microbiol 2003; 41(7): 2867-71.

[70]   Biswas D, Deb A, Gupta P, Prasad R, Negi KS. Evaluation of the usefulness of phage amplification technology in the diagnosis of patients with paucibacillary tuberculosis. Indian J Med Microbiol 2008; 26(1): 75-8.

[71]   Mbulo GM, Kambashi BS, Kinkese J, *et al.* Comparison of two bacteriophage tests and nucleic acid amplification for the diagnosis of pulmonary tuberculosis in sub-Saharan Africa. Int J Tuberc Lung Dis 2004; 8(11): 1342-7.

[72]   Mole R, Trollip A, Abrahams C, Bosman M, Albert H. Improved contamination control for a rapid phage-based rifampicin resistance test for *Mycobacterium tuberculosis*. J Med Microbiol 2007; 56(10): 1334-9.

[73]   Gali N, Dominguez J, Blanco S, *et al.* Use of a mycobacteriophage-based assay for rapid assessment of susceptibilities of *Mycobacterium tuberculosis* isolates to isoniazid and influence of resistance level on assay performance. J Clin Microbiol 2006; 44(1): 201-5.

[74]   Simboli N, Takiff H, McNerney R, *et al.* In-house phage amplification assay is a sound alternative for detecting rifampin-resistant *Mycobacterium tuberculosis* in low-resource settings. Antimicrob Agents Chemother 2005; 49(1): 425-7.

[75]   Traore H, Ogwang S, Mallard K, *et al.* Low-cost rapid detection of rifampicin resistant tuberculosis using bacteriophage in Kampala, Uganda. Ann Clin Microbiol Antimicrob 2007; 6(1): 1-3.

[76]   Chan ED, Heifets L, Iseman MD. Immunologic diagnosis of tuberculosis: A review. Tuber Lung Dis 2000; 80(3): 131-40.

[77]   Hillemann D, Rusch-Gerdes S, Richter E. Application of the Capilia TB assay for culture confirmation of *Mycobacterium tuberculosis* complex isolates. Int J Tuberc Lung Dis 2005; 9(12): 1409-11.

[78]   Fabre M, Gerome P, Maslin J, *et al.* Assessment of the Patho-TB kit for diagnosis of tuberculosis. Pathol Biol (Paris) 2007; 55(10): 482-5.

[79]   Pottumarthy S, Wells VC, Morris AJ. A comparison of seven tests for serological diagnosis of tuberculosis. J Clin Microbiol 2000; 38(6): 2227-31.

[80]   Abe C, Hirano K, Tomiyama T. Simple and rapid identification of the *Mycobacterium tuberculosis* complex by immunochromatographic assay using anti-MPB64 monoclonal antibodies. J Clin Microbiol 1999; 37(11): 3693-7.

[81]   Oettinger T, Andersen AB. Cloning and B-cell-epitope mapping of MPT64 from *Mycobacterium tuberculosis* H37Rv. Infect Immun 1994; 62(5): 2058-64.

[82]   Wang Z, Potter BM, Gray AM, Sacksteder KA, Geisbrecht BV, Laity JH. The solution structure of antigen MPT64 from *Mycobacterium tuberculosis* defines a new family of beta-grasp proteins. J Mol Biol 2007; 366(2): 375-81.

[83]   Guenin-Mace L, Simeone R, Demangel C. Lipids of pathogenic mycobacteria: Contributions to virulence and host immune suppression. Transbound Emerg Dis 2009; 56: 6-7.

[84]   Reither K, Saathoff E, Jung J, Minja LT, Kroidl I, Saad E, *et al.* Low sensitivity of a urine LAM-ELISA in the diagnosis of pulmonary tuberculosis. BMC Infect Dis 2009; 9: 141-2.

[85]   Boehme C, Molokova E, Minja F, Geis S, Loscher T, Maboko L, *et al.* Detection of Mycobacterial Lipoarabinomannan with an antigen-capture ELISA in unprocessed urine of Tanzanian patients with suspected tuberculosis. Trans R Soc Trop Med Hyg 2005; 99(12): 893-900.

[86]   Tessema TA, Hamasur B, Bjune G, Svenson S, Bjorvatn B. Diagnostic evaluation of urinary lipoarabinomannan at an Ethiopian tuberculosis centre. Scand J Infect Dis 2001; 33(4): 279-84.

[87]   Shah M, Variava E, Holmes CB, *et al.* Diagnostic accuracy of a urine lipoarabinomannan test for tuberculosis in hospitalized patients in a High HIV prevalence setting. J Acquir Immune Defic Syndr 2009; 52(2): 145-51.

[88]   Lawn SD, Edwards DJ, Kranzer K, Vogt M, Bekker LG, Wood R. Urine Lipoarabinomannan assay for tuberculosis screening before antiretroviral therapy diagnostic yield and association with immune reconstitution disease. AIDS 2009; 23(14): 1875-80.

[89]   Mathai E, Rajkumari R, Kuruvilla PJ, *et al.* Evaluation of serological tests for the diagnosis of tuberculosis. Indian J Pathol Bacteriol 2002; 45(3): 303-5.

[90]   Okuda Y, Maekura R, Hirotani A, *et al.* Rapid serodiagnosis of active pulmonary *Mycobacterium tuberculosis* by analysis of results from multiple antigen-specific tests. J Clin Microbiol 2004; 42(3): 1136-41.

[91]   Anderson BL, Welch RJ, Litwin CM. Assessment of three commercially available serologic assays for detection of antibodies to *Mycobacterium tuberculosis* and identification of active tuberculosis. Clin Vaccine Immunol 2008; 15(11): 1644-9.

[92]   Al-Hajjaj MS, Gad-El-Rab MO, Al-Orainey IO, Al-Kassimi FA. Improved sensitivity for detection of tuberculosis cases by a modified anda-TB ELISA test. Tuber Lung Dis. 1999; 79(3): 181-5.

[93]   Gupta S, Bhatia R, Datta KK. Serological diagnosis of childhood tuberculosis by estimation of mycobacterial antigen 60-specific immunoglobulins in the serum. Tuber Lung Dis. 1997; 78(1): 21-7.

[94]   Ghadiri K, Izadi B, Afsharian M, Vaziri Siavash R, Namdari S. Diagnostic value of serological tests (IgA, IgG, IgM) against A-60 antigen in tuberculosis. Iranian Journal of Clin Infect Dis 2008; 3(4): 205-8.

[95]   Kibiki GS, Mulder B, van der Ven AJ, *et al.* Laboratory diagnosis of pulmonary tuberculosis in TB and HIV endemic settings and the contribution of real time PCR for *M. tuberculosis* in bronchoalveolar lavage fluid. Trop Med Int Health 2007; 12(10): 1210-7.

[96]   Maekura R, Okuda Y, Nakagawa M, *et al.* Clinical evaluation of anti-tuberculous glycolipid immunoglobulin G antibody assay for rapid serodiagnosis of pulmonary tuberculosis. J Clin Microbiol 2001; 39(10): 3603-8.

[97] Steingart KR, Laal S, Hopewell PC, *et al.* Commercial serological antibody detection tests for the diagnosis of pulmonary tuberculosis: a systematic review. PLoS Med 2007; 4(6): 202.

[98] Steingart KR, Henry M, Laal S, *et al.* A systematic review of commercial serological antibody detection tests for the diagnosis of extrapulmonary tuberculosis. Postgrad Med J 2007; 83(985): 705-12.

[99] Lyashchenko K, Colangeli R, Houde M, Al Jahdali H, Menzies D, Gennaro ML. Heterogeneous antibody responses in tuberculosis. Infect Immun 1998; 66(8): 3936-40.

[100] Larsson S, Shrestha MP, Pokhrel BM, Upadhyay MP, Shrestha KB. The Glutaraldehyde test as a rapid screening method for pulmonary tuberculosis: a preliminary report. Ann Trop Med Parasitol 1990; 84(2): 111-7.

[101] Alavi-Naini R, Hashemi M, Mohagegh-Montazeri M, Sharifi-Mood B, Naderi M. Glutaraldehyde test for rapid diagnosis of pulmonary tuberculosis. Int J Tuberc Lung Dis 2009; 13(5): 601-5.

[102] Mathur ML, Sachdev R. Temperature affects the results of the glutaraldehyde test in the diagnosis of pulmonary tuberculosis. Int J Tuberc Lung Dis 2005; 9(2): 200-5.

[103] Mustafa AS, Amoudy HA, Wiker HG, *et al.* Comparison of antigen-specific T-cell responses of tuberculosis patients using complex or single antigens of *Mycobacterium tuberculosis*. Scand J Immunol 1998; 48(5): 535-43.

[104] Bhattacharyya S, Singla R, Dey AB, Prasad HK. Dichotomy of cytokine profiles in patients and high-risk healthy subjects exposed to tuberculosis. Infect Immun 1999; 67(11): 5597-603.

[105] Desem N, Jones SL. Development of a human gamma interferon enzyme immunoassay and comparison with tuberculin skin testing for detection of *Mycobacterium tuberculosis* infection. Clin Vaccine Immunol 1998; 5(4): 531-6.

[106] Streeton JA, Desem N, Jones SL. Sensitivity and specificity of a gamma interferon blood test for tuberculosis infection. Int J Tuberc Lung Dis 1998; 2(6): 443-50.

[107] Lalvani A, Pareek M. Interferon gamma release assays: Principles and practice. Enferm Infecc Microbiol Clin 2009; doi: 10.1016/j.eimc.2009.05.012.

[108] Machado AJ, Emodi K, Takenami I, *et al.* Analysis of discordance between the tuberculin skin test and the interferon-gamma release assay. Int J Tuberc Lung Dis 2009; 13(4): 446-53.

[109] Goletti D, Carrara S, Butera O, *et al.* Accuracy of immunodiagnostic tests for active tuberculosis using single and combined results: a multicenter TBNET-Study. PLoS One 2008; 3(10): 3417-8.

[110] Diel R, Loddenkemper R, Meywald-Walter K, Niemann S, Nienhaus A. Predictive value of a whole blood IFN-gamma assay for the development of active tuberculosis disease after recent infection with *Mycobacterium tuberculosis*. Am J Respir Crit Care Med 2008 ; 177(10): 1164-70.

[111] Nienhaus A, Schablon A, Diel R. Interferon-gamma release assay for the diagnosis of latent TB infection-analysis of discordant results, when compared to the tuberculin skin test. PLoS One 2008; 3(7): e2665.

[112] Kobashi Y, Mouri K, Obase Y, Fukuda M, Miyashita N, Oka M. Clinical evaluation of QuantiFERON TB-2G test for immunocompromised patients. Eur Respir J 2007; 30(5): 945-50.

[113] Winje BA, Oftung F, Korsvold GE, *et al.* School based screening for tuberculosis infection in Norway: comparison of positive tuberculin skin test with interferon-gamma release assay. BMC Infect Dis 2008; 8(1): 140-1.

[114] Ljghter J, Rigaud M, Eduardo R, Peng C, Pollack H. Latent tuberculosis diagnosis in children by using the QuantiFERON-TB Gold In-Tube test. Pediatrics 2009; 123(1): 30-7.

[115] Dosanjh DP, Hinks TS, Innes JA, *et al.* Improved diagnostic evaluation of suspected tuberculosis. Ann Intern Med 2008; 148(5): 325-36.

[116] Kang YA, Lee HW, Hwang SS, *et al.* Usefulness of whole-blood interferon-gamma assay and interferon-gamma enzyme-linked immunospot assay in the diagnosis of active pulmonary tuberculosis. Chest 2007; 132(3): 959-65.

[117] Kik SV, Franken WP, Arend SM, *et al.* Interferon-gamma release assays in immigrant contacts and effect of remote exposure to *Mycobacterium tuberculosis*. Int J Tuberc Lung Dis 2009; 13(7): 820-8.

[118] Janssens J, Roux-Lombard P, Perneger T, Metzger M, Vivien R, Rochat T. Contribution of a IFN-gamma assay in contact tracing for tuberculosis in a low-incidence, high immigration area. Swiss Med Wkly 2008; 138(39-40): 585-93.

[119] Porsa E, Cheng L, Graviss EA. Comparison of an ESAT-6/CFP-10 peptide-based enzyme-linked immunospot assay to a tuberculin skin test for screening of a population at moderate risk of contracting tuberculosis. Clin Vaccine Immunol 2007; 14(6): 714-9.

[120] Kobashi Y, Sugiu T, Shimizu H, *et al.* Clinical evaluation of the T-SPOT. TB test for patients with indeterminate results on the QuantiFERON TB-2G test. Intern Med 2009; 48(3): 137-42.

[121] Bakir M, Millington KA, Soysal A, *et al.* Prognostic value of a T-cell-based, interferon-gamma biomarker in children with tuberculosis contact. Ann Intern Med 2008; 149(11): 777-87.

[122] Thomas MM, Hinks TS, Raghuraman S, *et al.* Rapid diagnosis of *Mycobacterium tuberculosis* meningitis by enumeration of cerebrospinal fluid antigen-specific T-cells. Int J Tuberc Lung Dis 2008; 12(6): 651-7.

[123] World Health Organization. Guidance for National Tuberculosis Programs on the Management of Tuberculosis in Children. 2006. Report No. 2006.

[124] Marais BJ, Schaaf HS. Childhood tuberculosis: an emerging and previously neglected problem. Infect Dis Clin North Am 2010; 24(3): 727-49.

[125] Abu-Raddad LJ, Sabatelli L, Achterberg JT, *et al.* Epidemiological benefits of more-effective tuberculosis vaccines, drugs, and diagnostics. Proc Natl Acad Sci USA 2009; 106(33): 13980-5.

CHAPTER 8

Perspectives of Tuberculosis Management in Pediatric Disease

Selma M.A. Sias[1], Clemax C. Sant'Anna[2] and Paulo R.Z. Antas[3,*]

[1]Hospital Universitário Antônio Pedro, Universidade Federal Fluminense, Niterói, Brazil, [2]Universidade Federal do Rio de Janeiro, Rio de Janeiro, Brazil; Member of the Childhood Tuberculosis Group Stop TB initiative of the World Health Organization and [3]Laboratório de Imunologia Clínica, Fiocruz, Av. Brasil, # 4365; zip: 21045-900, Rio de Janeiro, Brazil

Abstract: Despite the lack of attention paid by effective control programs, childhood tuberculosis still remains an important public health problem. Identifying and treating tuberculosis infection and disease in children can also provide long-term benefits to tuberculosis control, preventing future cases due to reactivation. Rates of childhood tuberculosis appear to be rising, particularly in countries with generalized HIV epidemics. Data on childhood tuberculosis treatment outcomes is scarce. Unfortunately, measuring the true burden of childhood tuberculosis in any country is extremely difficult, because no diagnostic test performs well in childhood tuberculosis. Thus, in 25%-50% of childhood tuberculosis the tuberculin skin test may be invariably negative and, hence, much more progress needs to be made in obtaining better and faster diagnostic methods. Thus, perspectives at a management level are briefly described in this chapter in order to provide an update regarding recent advances in diagnosing tuberculosis.

Key Words: Tuberculosis, Children, Treatment, Antibiotic, Side Effects.

8.1. BACKGROUND

Tuberculosis remains a major public health problem worldwide, particularly in developing countries. The overall plan of the World Health Organization (WHO) "Stop TB Strategy" aims:

- To provide access to diagnostic detection of at least 70% of new cases and cure at least 85% of them.

- Promote the reduction of tuberculosis incidence and mortality rates by 50% by 2015.

- Eliminate the disease as a major public health problem by 2050.

It is well known that the tuberculosis situation became much worse in the HIV pandemic era, (one third of HIV patients are co-infected with *Mycobacterium tuberculosis*), and the emergence of drug-resistant strains of *M. tuberculosis* [1].

The absence of early diagnosis, the lack of sensitive tools to diagnose *M. tuberculosis* especially in HIV-infected patients, and the treatment of patients with active tuberculosis being not effective, particularly those with drug-resistant strains, are elements that still hinder the worldwide control of the disease [2, 3].

The outlook in the childhood population is no different. The low sensitivity and specificity of clinical and laboratory diagnosis of tuberculosis, associated with difficulty in obtaining biological samples for microbiological confirmation, plus the fact that in children bacilli in the respiratory secretions are sparse are key factors that hamper the diagnosis of tuberculosis in the pediatric population.

Tuberculosis in children is often diagnosed during routine assessment by means of contact survey focused on pulmonary tuberculosis patients. The positive tuberculin skin test (TST) result, plus the absence of

Address correspondence to Paulo R.Z. Antas: Laboratório de Imunologia Clínica, Fiocruz, Av. Brasil, # 4365; zip: 21045-900, Rio de Janeiro, Brazil; Tel: +55 21 3865-8152; E-mail: pzuquim@ioc.fiocruz.br

symptoms during physical examination and no radiologic abnormalities, defines latent tuberculosis infection (LTBI). When the contact child is symptomatic, tuberculosis enters in the differential diagnosis along with other common diseases, this is when epidemiological history and chest X-rays help the clinical diagnosis of active tuberculosis. However, the lack of epidemiological history of contact with tuberculosis adults does not rule out the diagnosis of tuberculosis in children.

In the majority of cases, the diagnosis of tuberculosis in children is not bacteriologically confirmed. Very frequently, the child under 5-years of age is paucibacillary, thus, the diagnostic criteria should be considered for epidemiological, clinical and radiological findings to establish the case identification [4]. In Brazil, the Ministry of Health scoring criteria, considering the clinical and radiologic characteristics, the contact history, as well as the TST and nutritional status of children, have been validated with high sensitivity and specificity, both in HIV-negative and -positive patients, and this can facilitate the diagnosis of disease in children [4, 5].

In tuberculosis and HIV co-infected children, the diagnostic criteria are similar to those for uninfected ones. However, those with significant impairment of the immune system may have atypical clinical manifestations of tuberculosis, making the final diagnosis difficult [1].

It was recently reported that a particularity of tuberculosis in children is the association of genotype of mycobacteria and the phenotype of the disease. Hesseling and colleagues (2010) [6] studied the phenotype of tuberculosis in intra-and extra-thoracic samples in 392 children at the age of 2-years old, hospitalized with tuberculosis culture-confirmed, and showed that the Beijing and S genotypes were more frequently found in cultures of extra-thoracic tuberculosis, indicating the potential risk of spread of these strains.

Due to paucibacillary characteristics of tuberculosis, children are not considered an important source of infection, contributing little in disease transmission. However, the disease in the pediatric population takes part in morbidity and mortality rates, especially in endemic areas where it is probably under diagnosed. In addition, the child acts as a reservoir and may develop the disease later in life. These data confirm the importance of research that would speed up the diagnosis allowing early treatment of LTBI and tuberculosis disease [7].

The difficulty of early diagnosis, especially in children, has stimulated a series of studies involving enzyme-linked immunoassays: molecular approaches and detection of specific mycobacterial antigens; more sensitive and rapid culture techniques; the use of induced-sputum techniques, in order to obtain better samples, for the early detection of the organism; as well as studies of drug-resistance based on nucleic acid amplification tests (NAATs) [8-11].

In adults, there are reports of rapid and simple approaches such as described by Goh and colleagues (2010) [12] who used the nitrate reductase activity of *M. tuberculosis* in commercially available automated liquid culture systems. While the Dubrous and colleagues (2009) [13] study optimized the microscopic examination using the "lower-priced fluorescence microscopes" and achieved faster diagnosis. During childhood, methods involving the search for bacilli, have restricted utility, due to the reasons given above.

Interferon-Gamma Release Assay (IGRA), such as QuantiFERON®-TB Gold and T-SPOT®.*TB* have demonstrated high specificity when compared to TST to detect LTBI, particularly in infant Bacille Calmette-Guerin (BCG) vaccinated populations. Unfortunately, IGRA is not very sensitive for active disease, and so it should be highlighted that a limiting factor of these new methods is the lack of study in child population in those areas where tuberculosis is endemic. Furthermore, its high cost is prohibitive in developing countries, where incidence and prevalence of the disease is high [14-16].

The treatment regimen, for tuberculosis in children, is similar to that recommended for adults whereby there is a use of several combinations of bactericidal drugs. The aim is to combat the *M. tuberculosis* populations that might be involved in the tubercle lesion, rapidly reducing the population of bacilli and hindering the emergence of mutants, resistant strains.

The currently recommended and proposed treatment scheme, in Brazil, is that all regimens should be conducted under supervision, and should be initiated for all children, (under 10-years of age), diagnosed with active tuberculosis, when the scoring scheme is equal to or more than 40 points. If the score is equal to, or more than 30 points, the treatment may also be established by clinical criteria [4; 5]. For children, it is recommended the basic treatment in two main stages: the attack stage, employing three drugs during 2 months: Rifampicin (R = 10 mgkg^{-1}), Isoniazid (H = 10 mgkg^{-1}) and Pyrazinamide (Z = 35 mgkg^{-1}), and the maintenance phase, taking up two drugs (R and Z) for 4 months. During adolescence ($\geq$ 10-years of age), the basic scheme for treatment consists of four drugs, associating the Ethambutol (E = 20-25 mgkg^{-1}) during the attack stage. Thus, the attack stage scheme is RHZE during 2 months, and R and Z in the maintenance phase, in the following 4 months. The serious side effect to E is optical neuritis. It is a very rare condition and quite difficult to identify in young children. The E is a safe drug for children if used at a dose of 20 mg/kg/day^{-1}. The basic scheme is suitable for the new cases of pulmonary and extrapulmonary tuberculosis (except for tuberculous meningitis) and for all those cases of relapse and recurrence after dropping out (Tables **1** and **2**) [5].

Table 1. Basic Scheme for Tuberculosis Management in Children Less Than 10-Years Old Dose per day.

Treatment stage	Drug	Up to 20 kg	From 20 to 35 kg	From 35 to 45 kg	More than 45 kg
Attack Stage (2 months)	R*	10#	300	450	600
	H	10	200	300	400
	Z	35	1,000	1,500	2,000
Maintenance phase (4 months)	R	10	300	450	600
	H	10	200	300	400

Indicated to new cases of all forms of pulmonary and extrapulmonary tuberculosis, including HIV-positive. *R=Rifampicin; H=Isoniazid; Z=Pyrazinamide. #mgkgday^{-1}.

Table 2. Basic Scheme for Tuberculosis Management in Adults and Adolescents (10-Years Old or Higher).

Regimen	Drug	Weight	Dose	Months
Attack stage	RHZE*	From 20 to 35 kg	2 pills	2
		From 36 to 50 kg	3 pills	
		More than 50 kg	4 pills	
Maintenance phase	RH	From 20 to 35 kg	1 pill (or 300/200 mg)	4
		From 36 to 50 kg	1 pill (or 300/200 mg) + 1 pill (or 150/100 mg)	
		More than 50 kg	2 pills (or 300/200 mg)	

*R=Rifampicin; H=Isoniazid; Z=Pyrazinamide; E=Ethambutol.

For tuberculous meningitis cases, the total time of treatment is 9 months (2 months of attack stage, and 7 months of maintenance phase). It should be associated with steroids (prednisone = 1-2 mgkgday^{-1} for 4 weeks, or in severe cases dexamethasone = 0.3-0.4 mgkgday^{-1} for 4-8 weeks) with gradual decrease in 4 weeks following (Tables **3** and **4**) [5].

Table 3. Basic Scheme Suitable for Tuberculous Meningitis Management in Children Dose per day.

Treatment stage	Drug	Dose (all ages)	From 20 to 35 kg	From 35 to 45 kg	More than 45 kg
Attack Stage (2 months)	R*	10 to 20#	300	450	600
	H	10 to 20	200	300	400
	Z	35	1,000	1,500	2,000
Maintenance phase (7 months)	R	10 to 20	300	450	600
	H	10 to 20	200	300	400

Indicated to: (a) cases of concomitant tuberculous meningitis and any given location, (b) in tuberculous meningitis, it should be associated to steroids and anti-tuberculosis regimen (oral prednisone [1-2 mgkgday^{-1}] for 4 weeks or intra-venous dexamethasone in severe cases [0.3-0.4 mgkgday^{-1}] for 4-8 weeks, gradual dose reduction afterwards), and (c) the physical therapy in tuberculous meningitis should be initiated as soon as possible. *R=Rifampicin; H=Isoniazid; Z=Pyrazinamide. #mgkgday^{-1}.

Table 4. Basic Scheme for Meningoencephalitis Tuberculosis Management in Adults and Adolescents (10-Years Old or Higher).

Regimen	Drug	Weight	Dose	Months
Attack stage	RHZE*	35 kg From 36 to 50 kg More than 50 kg	2 pills 3 pills 4 pills	2
Maintenance phase	RH	35 kg From 36 to 50 kg More than 50 kg	1 pill (or 300/200 mg) 1 pill (or 300/200 mg) + 1 pill (or 150/100 mg) 2 pills (or 300/200 mg)	7

Indicated to: (a) cases of concomitant tuberculous meningitis and any given location, tuberculous meningitis scheme use, (b) in tuberculous meningitis, it should be associated to steroids and anti-tuberculosis regimen (oral prednisone [1-2 mgkgday^{-1}] for 4 weeks or intra-venous dexamethasone in severe cases [0.3-0.4 mgkgday^{-1}] for 4-8 weeks, gradual dose reduction afterwards), and (c) the physical therapy in tuberculous meningitis should be initiated as soon as possible. *R=Rifampicin; H=Isoniazid; Z=Pyrazinamide; E=Ethambutol.

Little is known about multidrug-resistant (MDR) tuberculosis in the pediatric population. The child contact with a MDR tuberculosis case, or coming from regions with high rate of primary MDR tuberculosis (more than 4%), is likely to be infected with the same resistant strain and is also vulnerable to develop the tuberculosis disease. The selection and spread of MDR *M. tuberculosis* strains constitute a major threat to global tuberculosis control. Since the emergence of these strains is mainly associated with treatment noncompliance, a strategy suggested by WHO is the Directly Observed Treatment Short Course (DOTS), thus ensuring the effective treatment of patients with active tuberculosis and breaking the transmission chain. In Brazil, after a partial implementation of the DOTS strategy, there has been a 26% drop in tuberculosis incidence and a 32% reduction in mortality rates; therefore, it seems a promising strategy [1, 3, 5].

In the majority of cases, the antimicrobial treatment for tuberculosis is well tolerated by a given child, without any significant adverse effect. Side effects are quite rare although they do occur more frequently in malnourished children with a prior history of liver disease, as well as those with advanced HIV disease. Side effects are classified into major and minor ones. Those categorized as minor are:

- Anorexia.
- Nausea.
- Vomiting.
- Abdominal pain (RHZ).
- Pruritus (RS).
- Joint pain (Z).
- Paresthesia.
- Euphoria.
- Insomnia.
- Anxiety.
- Drowsiness and headache (H).
- Red or orange colored urine.
- Sweat (R).

Generally, treatment is symptomatic; there is no need to stop anti-tuberculosis drugs. On the other hand, the major effects are:

- Seizure (H).

- Hearing loss.

- Vertigo.

- Nystagmus (S).

- Optical neuritis (E).

- Systemic reaction.

- Shock.

- Purpura (R).

- Rash/pruritus (RS).

- Encephalopathy.

- Jaundice (HRZE).

- Hepatitis

The major side effects should be carefully evaluated in case of medical attention is needed; for more severe forms, hospitalization is suggested. The first-line drugs (RHZ) may cause liver damage (hepatitis induced by drugs) but R can cause jaundice, without hepatitis evidence [1].

There are no standardized therapeutic regimens for the use in childhood cases of MDR tuberculosis. Whenever possible, the scheme for the child (which is usually paucibacillary) should be based on susceptibility testing of the index case [1].

Patients co-infected with *M. tuberculosis* and HIV represent another challenge and require early initiation of antiretroviral treatment, since it is well known that HIV-infected children are at greater risk of developing more severe forms. There is still no consensus on the management of these cases, but the preventive therapy is an important approach in contacts with high risk of MDR tuberculosis [7, 17].

In those cases with suspected tuberculosis plus severe immunosuppressed individuals, empirical tuberculosis treatment should be instituted during the still pending laboratory tests. In adolescent and adult cases, it might always be recommended the culture associated to the susceptibility testing, because of higher prevalence, in these patients, of infection with non-tuberculous mycobacteria and higher incidence of MDR tuberculosis. In those patients co-infected with *M. tuberculosis* and HIV they should be given priority to tuberculosis treatment and, when indicated, initiate antiretroviral therapy 2 to 4 weeks after initiation of tuberculosis treatment [5].

Some tuberculosis and HIV co-infected children with significant impairment of immunity, (usually with CD4 T lymphocyte count lower than 15%), may present after initiation of potent antiretroviral therapy, the Immune Reconstitution Inflammatory Syndrome (IRIS), a significant inflammatory reaction in places where *M. tuberculosis* is present. This syndrome follows with exacerbation or reemergence of tuberculosis, exacerbation of pre-conditions such as dermatitis, fever, weight loss, lymph node enlargements, abscess at the site of BCG vaccination after years, consolidation, and pleural effusion. The occurrence of IRIS does not change the treatment regimen for tuberculosis, but in some instances it should be associated with steroids in severe cases. The incidence of IRIS is higher in patients with opportunistic infections before antiretroviral therapy [5, 18].

Another concern related to tuberculosis and HIV co-infected patients is the adverse drug interactions with anti-tuberculosis therapy, occurring between 18-42% of cases. It is often necessary to change the course of treatment and requires a close monitoring scheme and clinical and laboratory vigilance, enhancing the treatment cost and increasing the likelihood of dropping out. Rifampicin has been marked as the most frequent drug implicated with the onset of side effects. Rifabutin is an effective alternative therapy allowing simultaneous use with antiretroviral drugs as Indinavir, Nelfinavir and Amprenavir in adults [19].

New therapeutic regimens that stimulate the immune system such as interleukin-2, interleukin 12, interferon-gamma and antagonists of tumor necrosis factor have been tested with promising results [2, 19].

Innovative experimental research related to gene therapy has also been developed. Lorenzi and colleagues (2010) [20] developed an experimental vaccine with mRNA of *M. leprae* hsp65 protein intranasally delivered and capable of conferring protection against virulent *M. tuberculosis*, thus expanding new perspective in chemoprophylaxis.

Besides the treatment of active tuberculosis, another important strategy in disease control is the early detection and treatment of LTBI in infected individuals with a higher risk of progression to active disease. Individuals with LTBI are at greater risk of developing tuberculosis disease, particularly in the first 2 years after infection, with approximately 90% of cases occurring among contacts during this period [5, 11].

In Brazil, children with LTBI are detected by the TST reaction after the clearance (clinical and radiological) of tuberculosis disease [5]. The cutoff for TST currently used in Brazil is 5 mm, considering that the recent contacts equal to or more than 12-years of age, and HIV-negative, have a 6-fold risk to acquire LTBI, when compared to those with TST less than 5 mm; treatment for LTBI is indicated in the following cases:

- *TST ≥ 5 mm* = co-infected *M. tuberculosis* and HIV patients, recent contacts (less than 2 years) of pulmonary tuberculosis and BCG-vaccinated for more than 2 years, untreated tuberculosis patients with radiological lung sequel at chest X-ray, grafted and transplant candidates, other cases of immunosuppressed individuals, such as prolonged use of steroids (prednisone ≥ 15 mgday^{-1} or equivalent for more than 1 month) and blocking tumor necrosis factor treatment.

- *Recent TST conversion* (≥ 10 mm when performed between 2 weeks and 2 years after previous TST) = workers in the prison system, caregivers for the elderly people, mycobacteria laboratory personnel, health professionals and recent contacts of pulmonary tuberculosis at any age.

- *TST ≥ 10 mm* = recent contacts (< 2 years) of pulmonary tuberculosis and BCG-vaccinated equal to or less 2 years, injecting-drug users, immunosuppressed patients (insulin-dependent diabetes mellitus, silicosis, lymphoma, cancer of the head, neck and lung, or other procedures, such as gastrectomy, hemodialysis and gastrointestinal bypass) and indigenous people.

- *Independent TST* = HIV-positive patients with a history of recent contact (< 2 years) with active pulmonary tuberculosis patients or radiographic image showing sequel of pulmonary tuberculosis with no previous history of tuberculosis treatment, disregard the TST score.

The drug used is Isoniazid (H = 5 to 10 mgkg^{-1} to 300 mgday^{-1}) for 6 months [5].

In special situations the newborn is managed as primary chemoprophylaxis; this occurs when the mother, or other relative, harbor the bacillus. Before BCG vaccination, it is initiated an administration of H for 3 months. Afterwards, the child should proceed to the TST. If it turns positive (≥ 5 mm), chemoprophylaxis must be maintained (until the sixth month); however if the TST remains negative (< 5 mm), the chemoprophylaxis may be suspended and then proceed to regular BCG vaccination [5].

The complications of tuberculosis in children are rare, although often involving the BCG vaccination; severe axillaries lymphadenitis, abscess, osteomyelitis and systemic spread. Furthermore. they can be as a result of primary tuberculosis, such as hilar or mediastinal lymphadenopathy, which can induce tracheobronchial tree compression resulting in atelectasis, ulceration, perforation and calcification. Santos and colleagues (2010) [21] underscore the importance of delaying the BCG vaccination in children, with a family history of primary immunodeficiency, until this condition is ruled out. This is due to an increased risk of severe complications in this group [22].

Endobronchial tuberculosis is a rare complication of primary tuberculosis in pediatric population and should always be investigated in children during tuberculosis treatment with signs or symptoms of airway obstruction. The diagnosis is usually delayed and may lead to atelectasis, bronchiectasis and scarring stenosis. Ledesma-Albarran and colleagues (1996) [23] performed bronchovideoscopy in 30 children with radiological changes. Those cases had chest X-rays segmental or lobular atelectasis, paratracheal or hilar lymphadenopathy, consolidation and localized hyperinflation, However in 36.6% of children with no evident clinical or radiological sign of tuberculosis. They found endobronchial tuberculosis. Then, the diagnostic confirmation of endobronchial tuberculosis is performed by bronchoscopy which can reveal changes, such as compression by adenopathy, mucosal erosion, granuloma, and caseous and polypoid lesions. These endoscopic changes justify, in most severe cases, a combination of steroids in an attempt to prevent stenosis [24-26].

8.2. TUBERCULOSIS AS AN OUT-OF-CONTROL PROBLEM

So far, tuberculosis diagnosis in endemic settings has gained little benefit from scientific progress by means of biotechnological developments [27]. Unfortunately, there is still an urgent demand for a field-friendly test, which would be able to diagnose tuberculosis on the spot in order to avoid delays in diagnosis, preventing further transmission and reducing complications. The ideal field diagnostics for tuberculosis should; be available in one hour, require no electricity, refrigeration, fresh water supply or highly trained personnel [28].

Strengthening rational surveillance to capture all diagnosed cases of tuberculosis in children will help provide more accurate estimates of disease burden and potentially increase political commitment to address childhood tuberculosis. Efforts should be geared towards diagnostic tuberculosis research in developing countries to facilitate early diagnosis of cases and prompt initiation of therapy for tuberculosis control program to have a meaningful impact in the community.

The plague of tuberculosis, a disease that has existed for over 8,000 years, is not only about the clinical diagnosis, prophylaxis and treatment regimens; it is in social involvement, including the civil society, governments, managers, universities and research centers. There is an urgent need for commitment, from all these sectors, to really achieve and embrace the objectives of the program. However, efforts should be geared towards diagnostic tuberculosis research, in developing countries, to facilitate early diagnosis of cases and prompt initiation of therapy for tuberculosis control programs; this will lead to a meaningful impact in the community.

Achieving a more efficient and accurate diagnosis of infection is an essential arm for the control of tuberculosis. The improvement in the detection rates, as well as the reduction in the time to correct management of the disease, will impact the duration of infectiousness, disease progression and severity, eventually contributing to a decreased mortality and transmission rate [29; 30].

REFERENCES

[1]   World Health Organization. Guidance for National Tuberculosis Programs on the Management of Tuberculosis in Children. 2006. Report No.: 2006.

[2]   Riccardi G, Pasca MR, Buroni S. *Mycobacterium tuberculosis*: drug resistance and future perspectives. Future Microbiol 2009; 4: 597-614.

[3]   Migliori GB, Centis R, Lange C, Richardson MD, Sotgiu G. Emerging epidemic of drug-resistant tuberculosis in Europe, Russia, China, South America and Asia: current status and global perspectives. Curr Opin Pulm Med 2010; 16(3): 171-9.

[4]   Pedrozo C, Sant'Anna CC, March MF, Lucena SC. Efficacy of the scoring system, recommended by the Brazilian National Ministry of Health, for the diagnosis of pulmonary tuberculosis in children and adolescents, regardless of their HIV status. J Bras Pneumol 2010; 36(1): 92-8.

[5]   III Brazilian Thoracic Association Guidelines on Tuberculosis. J Bras Pneumol 2009; 35(10): 1018-48.

[6]   Hesseling AC, Marais BJ, Kirchner HL, *et al.* Mycobacterial genotype is associated with disease phenotype in children. Int J Tuberc Lung Dis 2010; 14(10): 1252-8.

[7]   Marais BJ, Schaaf HS. Childhood tuberculosis: an emerging and previously neglected problem. Infect Dis Clin North Am 2010; 24(3): 727-49.

[8]   Zar HJ, Hanslo D, Apolles P, Swingler G, Hussey G. Induced sputum versus gastric lavage for microbiological confirmation of pulmonary tuberculosis in infants and young children: a prospective study. Lancet 2005; 365: 130-4.

[9]   van Hung N, Sy DN, Anthony RM, Cobelens FG, van Soolingen D. Fluorescence microscopy for tuberculosis diagnosis. Lancet Infect Dis 2007; 7(4): 238-9.

[10]   Martire TM. Diagnostico laboratorial da tuberculose na infancia: metodos convencionais e metodos rapidos. Pulmao RJ 2009; 20(1): 27-9.

[11]   Zar HJ, Connell TG, Nicol M. Diagnosis of pulmonary tuberculosis in children: new advances. Expert Rev Anti Infect Ther 2010; 8(3): 277-88.

[12]   Goh KS, Rasgoti N. Simple and rapid method for detection of nitrate reductase activity of *Mycobacterium tuberculosis* and *Mycobacterium canetti* grown in the Bactec MGIT960 system. J Microbiol Methods 2010; 81920: 208-10.

[13]   Dubrous P, Alaoui H, N'Dounga Mikolo B, Koeck JL. Diagnosis of tuberculosis in developing countries: new perspectives. Med Trop 2009; 69(6): 618-28.

[14]   Menzies D, Pai M, Comstock G. Meta-analysis: new tests for the diagnosis of latent tuberculosis infection: areas of uncertainty and recommendations for research. Ann Intern Med 2007 Mar 6; 146(5): 340-54.

[15]   Sztajnbok FR, Boechat NL, Sztajnbok DC, Ribeiro SB, Oliveira SK, Sant'Anna CC. The challenge of pediatric tuberculosis in face of new diagnostic techniques. J Ped 2009; 85(3): 183-93.

[16]   Tsolia MN, Mavrikou M, Critselis E, *et al.* Whole blood interferon-gamma release assay is a useful tool for the diagnosis of tuberculosis infection particularly among Bacille Calmette Guerin-vaccinated children. Pediatr Infect Dis J 2010; 29(12): 1137-40.

[17]   Shaaf HS, Marais BJ. Management of multidrug-resistant tuberculosis in children: a survival guide for paediatricians. Paediatr Respir Rev 2011; 12(1): 31-8.

[18]   Puthanakit T, Oberdorfer P, Punjaisee S, Wannarit P, Thira Sirisanthana T, Sirisanthana V. Immune Reconstitution Syndrome due to Bacillus Calmette-Guerin after initiation of antiretroviral therapy in children with HIV infection. Clin Infect Dis 2005; 41(7): 1049-52.

[19]   Anonimous. XI Virtual Congress HIV/AIDS TB. 2010. Report No.: 1.

[20]   Lorenzi JC, Trombone AP, Rocha CD, *et al.* Intranasal vaccination with messenger RNA as a new approach in gene therapy: use against tuberculosis. BMC Biotechnol 2010; 10: 77-8.

[21]   Santos A, Dias A, Cordeiro A, *et al.* Severe axillary lymphadenitis after BCG vaccination: alert for primary immunodeficiencies. J Microbiol Immunol Infect 2010; 43(6): 530-7.

[22]   Sadeghi-Shabestari M, Rezaei N. Disseminated bacille Calmette-Guerin in Iranian children with severe combined immunodeficiency. Int J Infect Dis 2009; 13(6): 420-3.

[23]   Ledesma Albarran JM, Perez Ruiz E, Fernandez V, Gonzalez Martinez B, Perez Frias J, Martinez Valverde A. Endoscopic evaluation of endobronchial tuberculosis in children. Arch Bronconeumol 1996; 32(4): 183-6.

[24]   Milward GA, Sias SMA, Zimmerman J, Ferreira AS, Pinho MA. Bronchoscopic findings in the tuberculosis in children. Eur Resp J 2000; 16(31): 482-3.

[25]   Prada Arias M, Jardon Bahia JA, Rodriguez Barca P, *et al.* Endobronchial tuberculous granuloma in children. Eur J Pediatr Surg 2006; 16(4): 265-8.

[26]   Cakir E, Uyan ZS, Oktem S, *et al.* Flexible bronchoscopy for diagnosis and follow up of childhood endobronchial tuberculosis. Pediatr Infect Dis J 2008; 27(9): 783-7.

[27]   Perkins MD, Roscigno G, Zumla A. Progress towards improved tuberculosis diagnostics for developing countries. Lancet 2006; 367: 942-3.

[28]   Keeler E, Perkins MD, Small P, *et al.* Reducing the global burden of tuberculosis: the contribution of improved diagnostics. Nature 2006; 444: 49-57.

[29]   Perkins MD, Cunningham J. Facing the crisis: improving the diagnosis of tuberculosis in the HIV era. J Infect Dis 2007; 196(1): 15-27.

[30]   Abu-Raddad LJ, Sabatelli L, Achterberg JT, *et al.* Epidemiological benefits of more-effective tuberculosis vaccines, drugs, and diagnostics. Proc Natl Acad Sci USA 2009; 106(33): 13980-5.

APPENDIX

A) X-RAY IMAGES

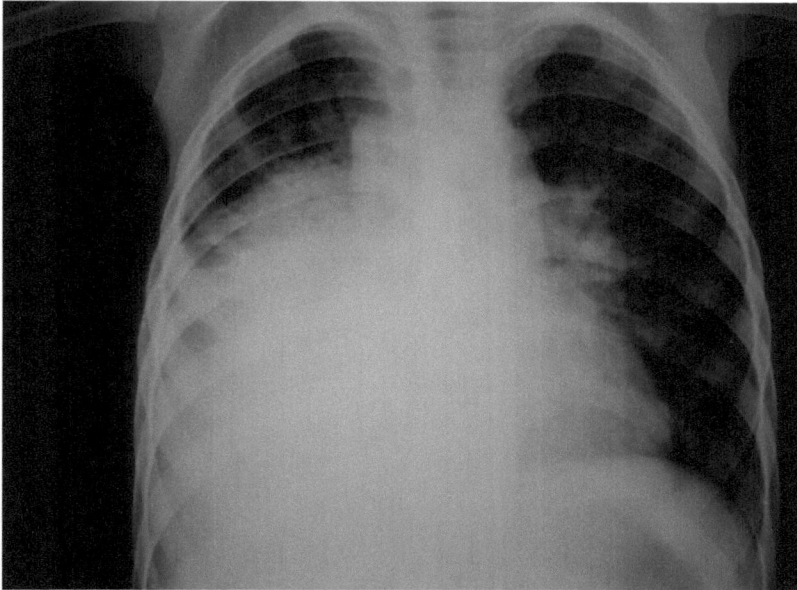

A girl with fever and persistent cough for 2 weeks was admitted in the emergency room where there was carried out chest X-ray due to the extensive pneumonia in the right lung. She was medicated as regular pneumonia, without clinical and radiological improvement. PPD was not reactor; erythrocyte sedimentation rate and C-Reactive Protein were high, but HIV test was negative. CT scan was also recorded (see below).

Source: Author.

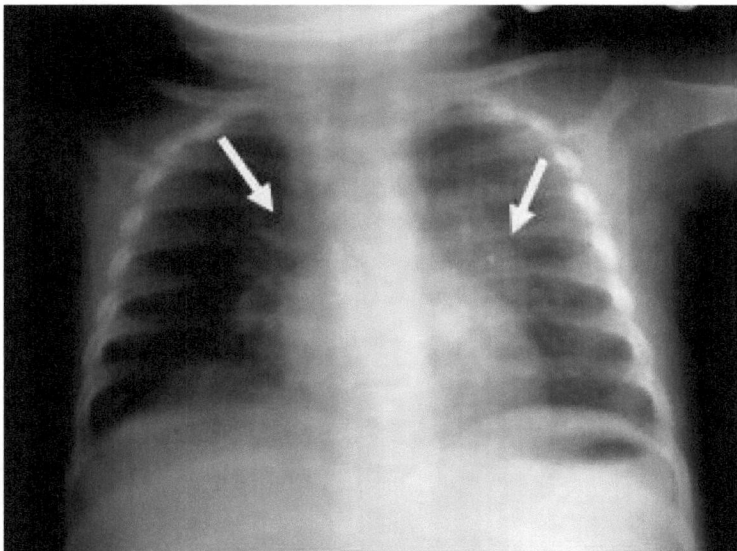

X-ray image of bilateral mediastinal enlargement (arrows) in a 6-months breastfeeding baby which was also household contact of an adult index case of tuberculosis. TST=15 mm.

Source: Author.

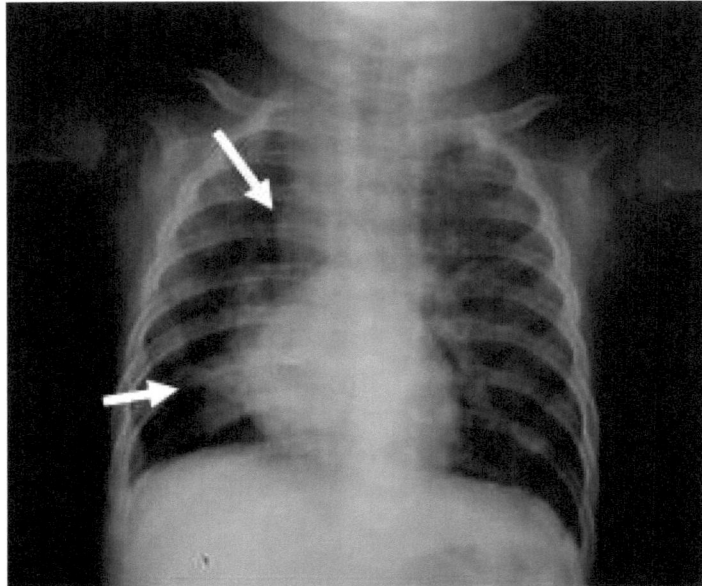

X-ray image showing right hilar and paratracheal lymphadenopathy (arrows) as a typical finding in childhood primary tuberculosis.

Source: Author.

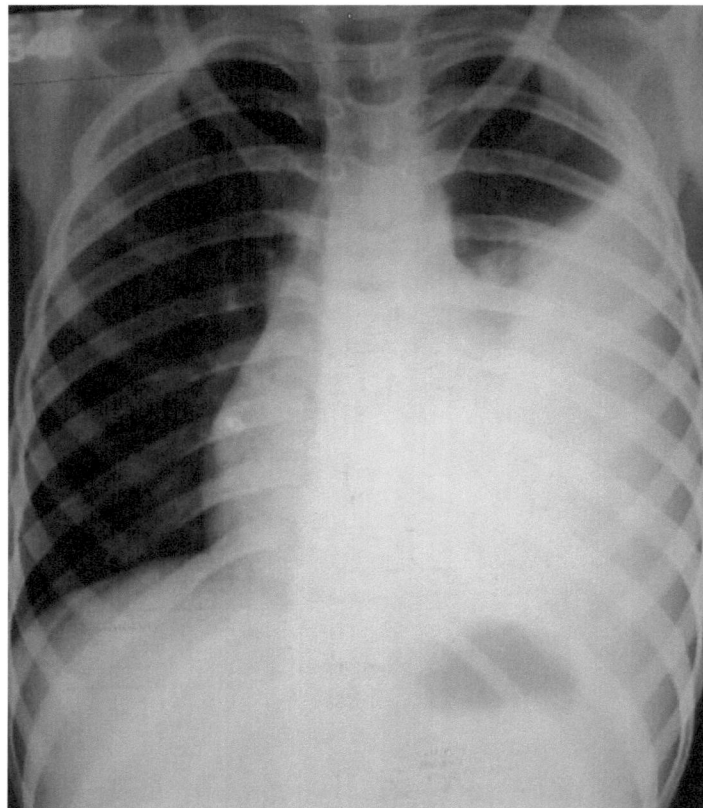

Chest X-ray image showing tuberculosis pleural effusion in 16-years old boy.

Source: Author.

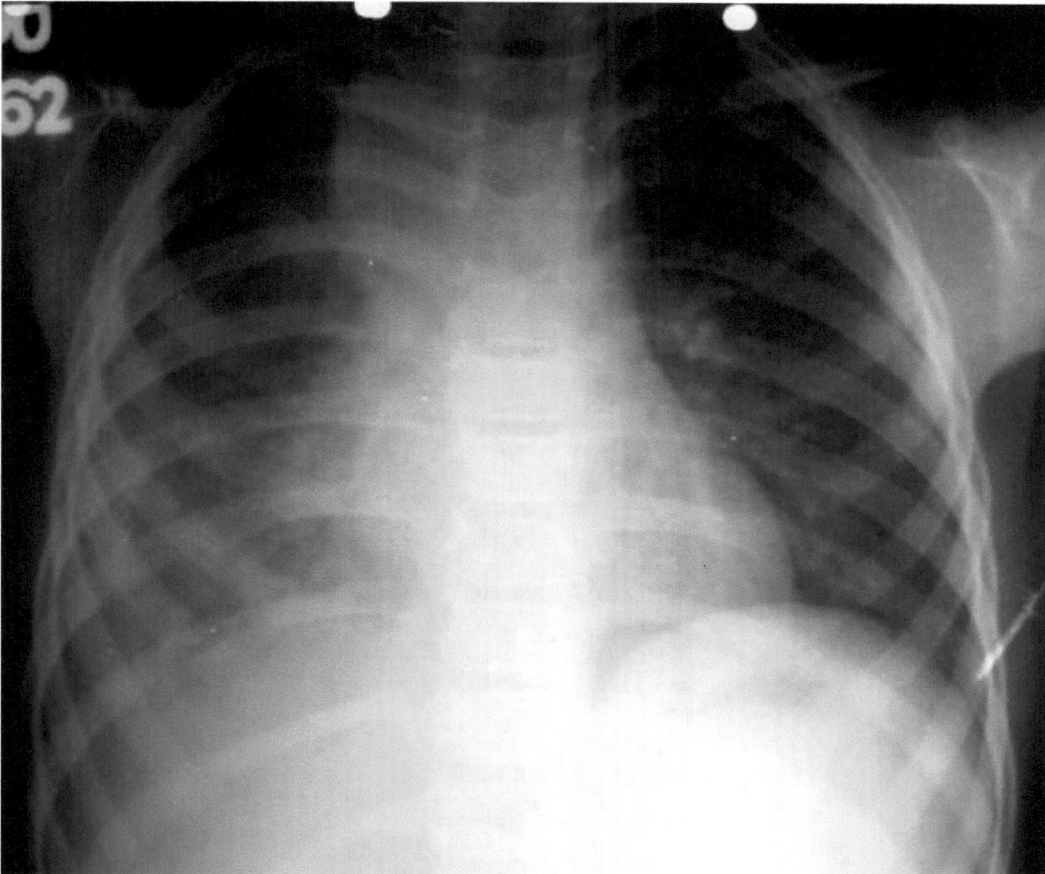

X-ray image showing right paratracheal lymphadenopathy, pleural effusion and airspace opacity in the right lower lobe in a HIV-positive 10-years old boy. The broncoalveolar lavage aspirate yielded culture-positive for *Mycobacterium tuberculosis*.

Source: Author.

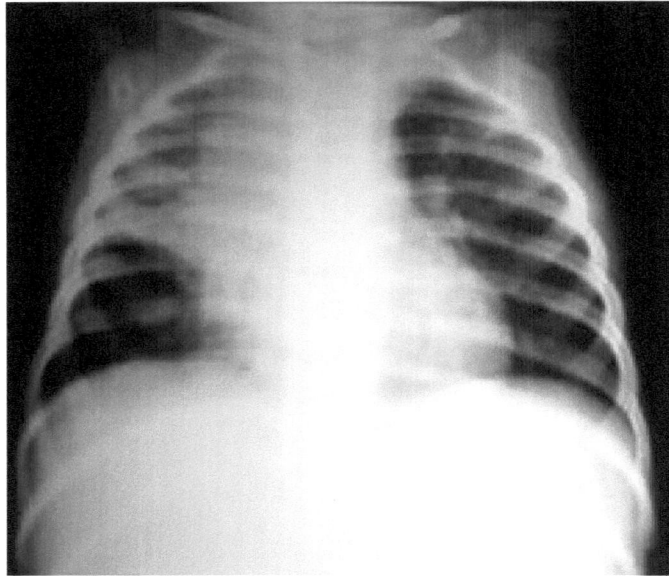

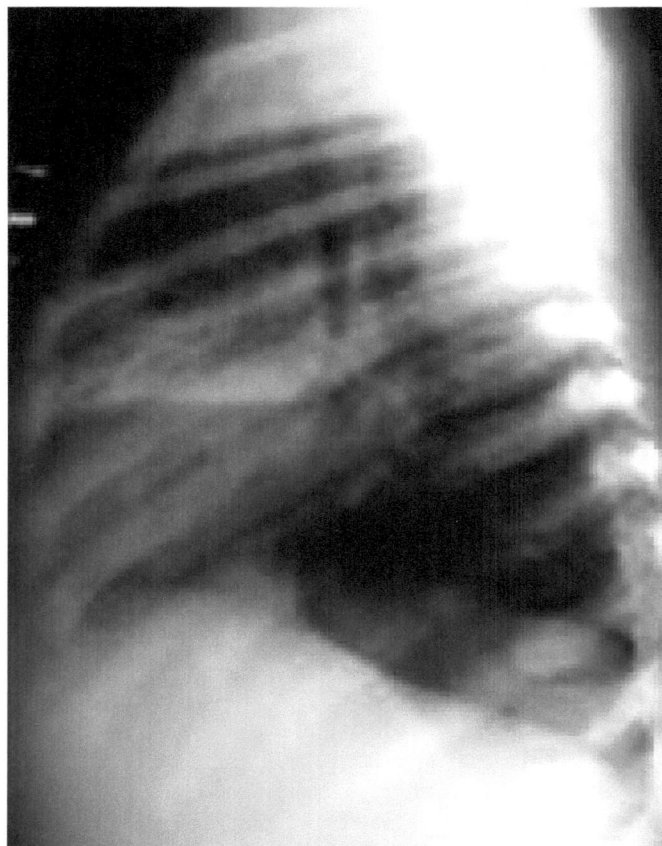

X-ray image of the right upper lobe collapse-consolidation lesion in a drug-resistant tuberculosis case of a 9-months breastfeeding and malnourished baby (Front and lateral view). The broncoalveolar lavage aspirate yielded culture-positive for *Mycobacterium tuberculosis*.

Source: Author.

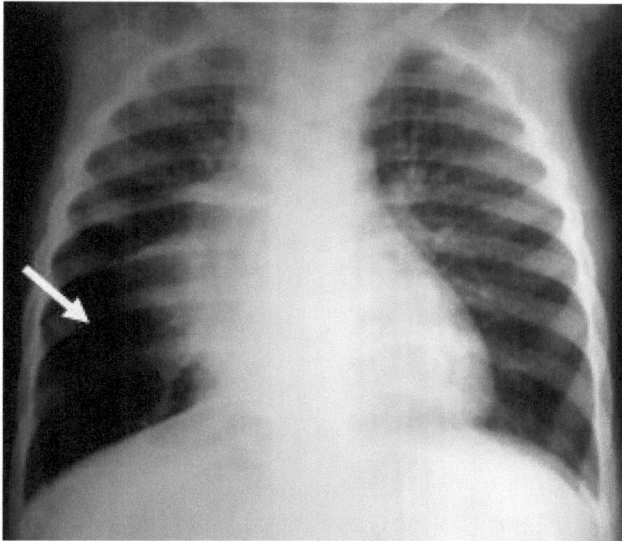

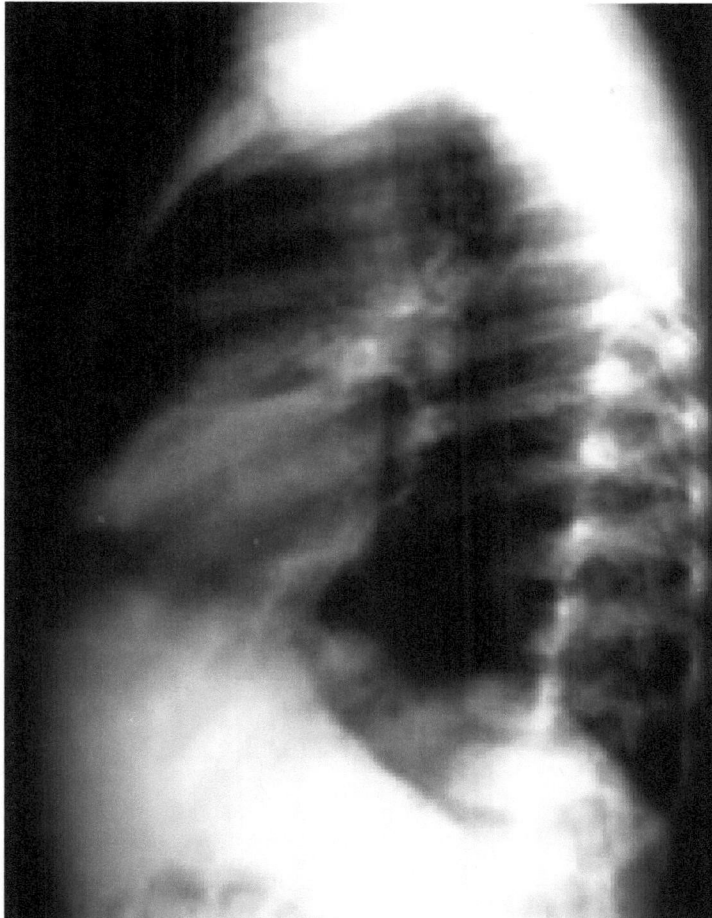

Another form of tuberculosis in children: localized hyperinflation (arrow) due to extrinsic compression of the bronchial lymph nodes (Front and lateral view).

Source: Author.

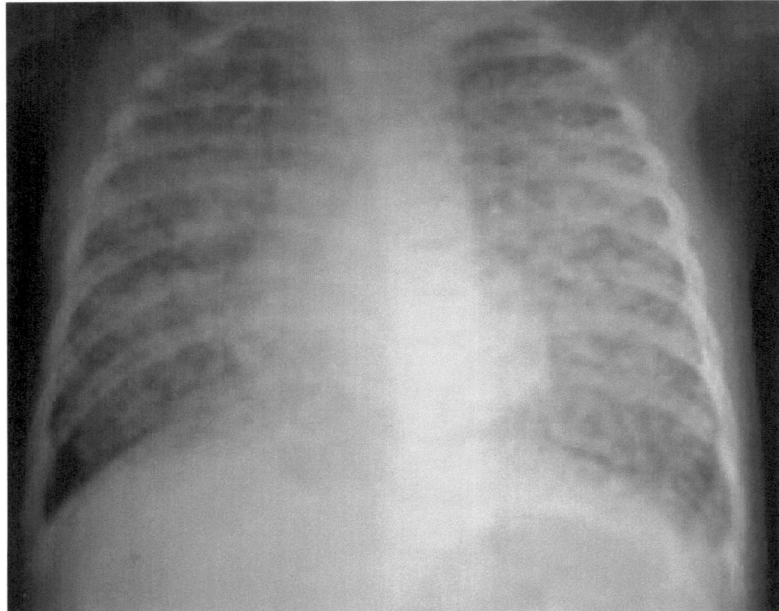

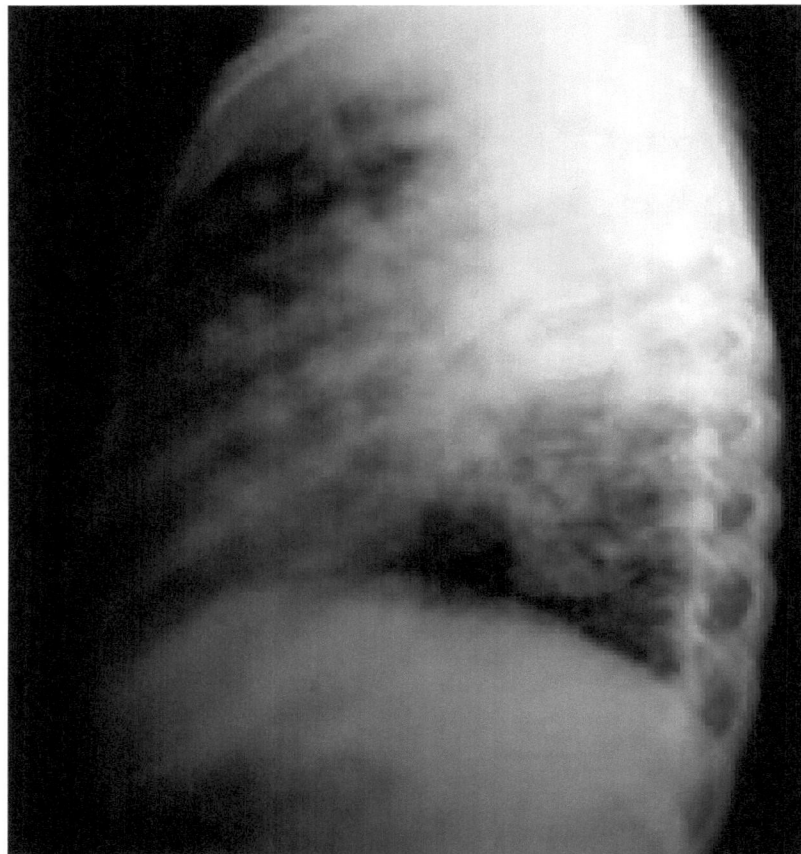

Chest X-ray image showing diffuse micronodular infiltration of both lungs in a newborn with miliary tuberculosis (Front and lateral view).

Source: Author.

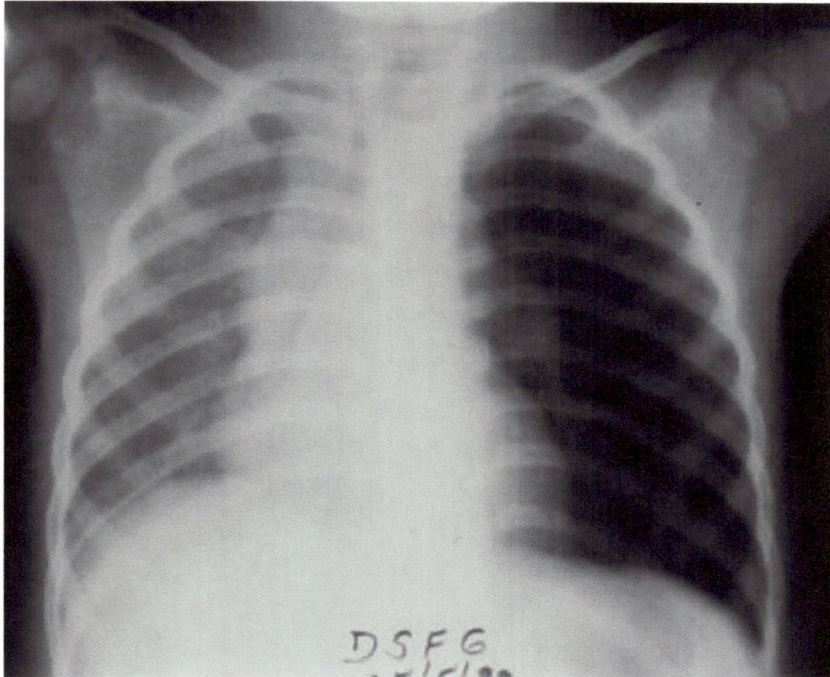

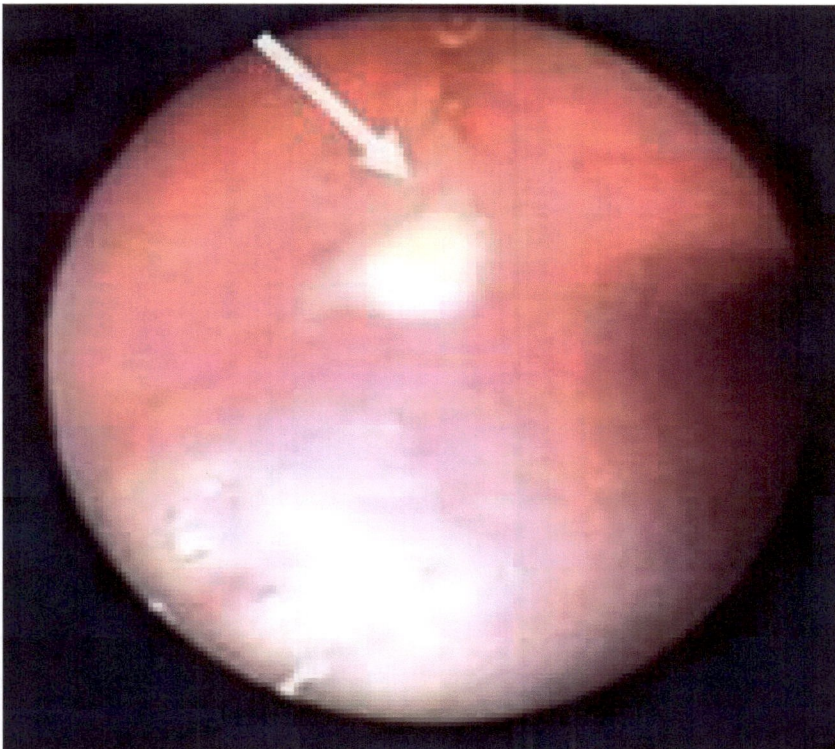

Top: Chest X-ray image of a 3-years old girl mimicking foreign body aspiration: hyperinflation due to extrinsic compression of the left main bronchus. Bottom: Broncoscopy image showing an extrinsic compression of the left main bronchus due to fistulae of lymph node into the bronchus.

Source: Author.

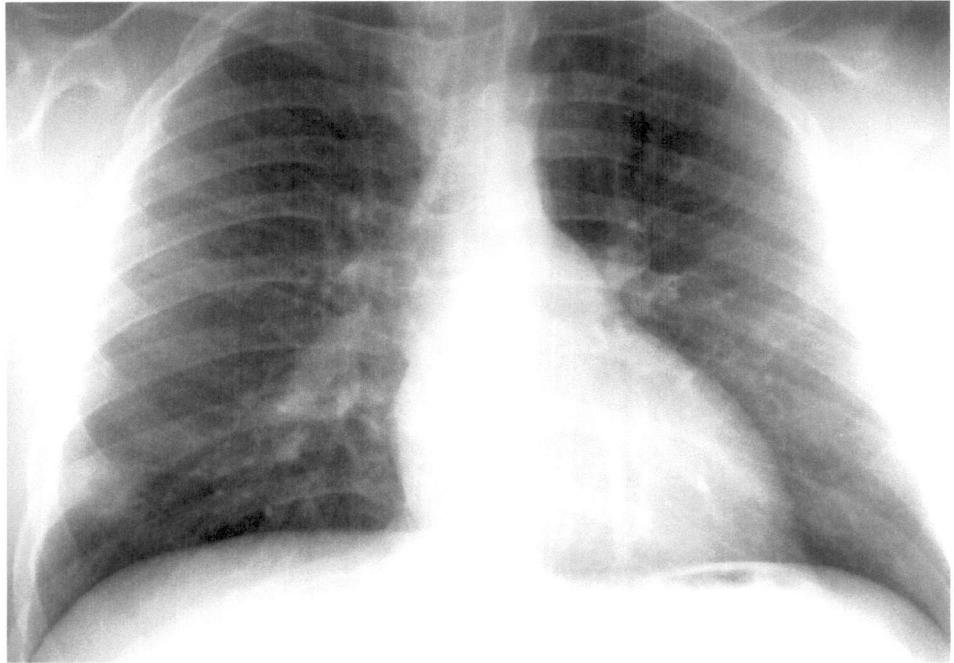

A peripheral airspace opacity in the right lower lobe and right hilar lymphadenopathy. This is an example of the primary complex (Ghon focus and ipsilateral hilar lymphadenopathy) that is typical of primary tuberculosis in a child.

Source: Francis J. Curry National Tuberculosis Center.

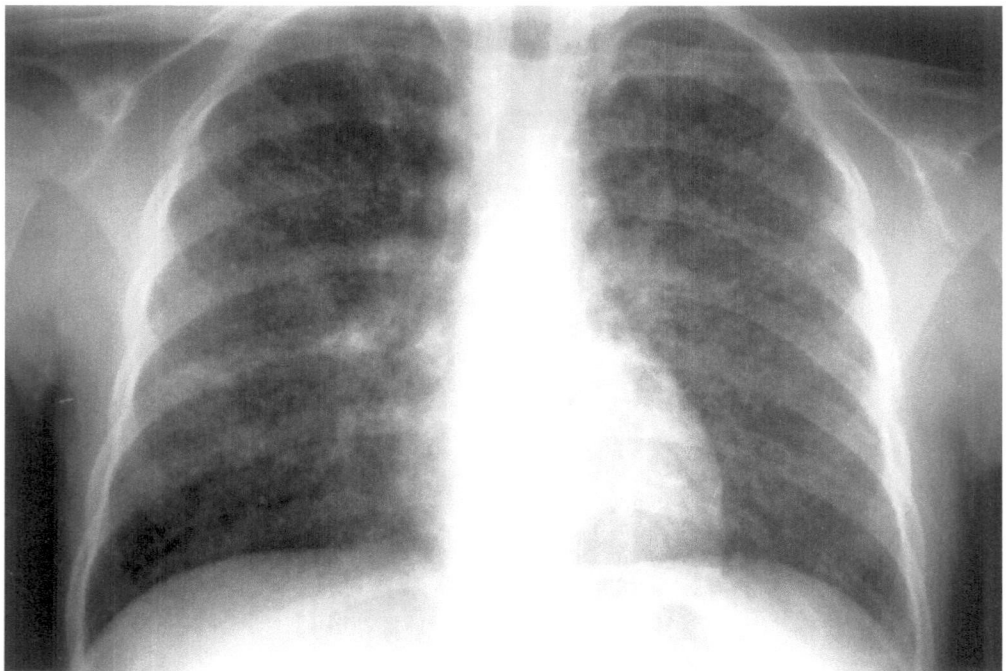

Bilateral diffuse small nodules (2-3 mm in diameter) consistent with a military pattern. The patient was a 5 years-old girl with disseminated tuberculosis.

Source: Francis J. Curry National Tuberculosis Center.

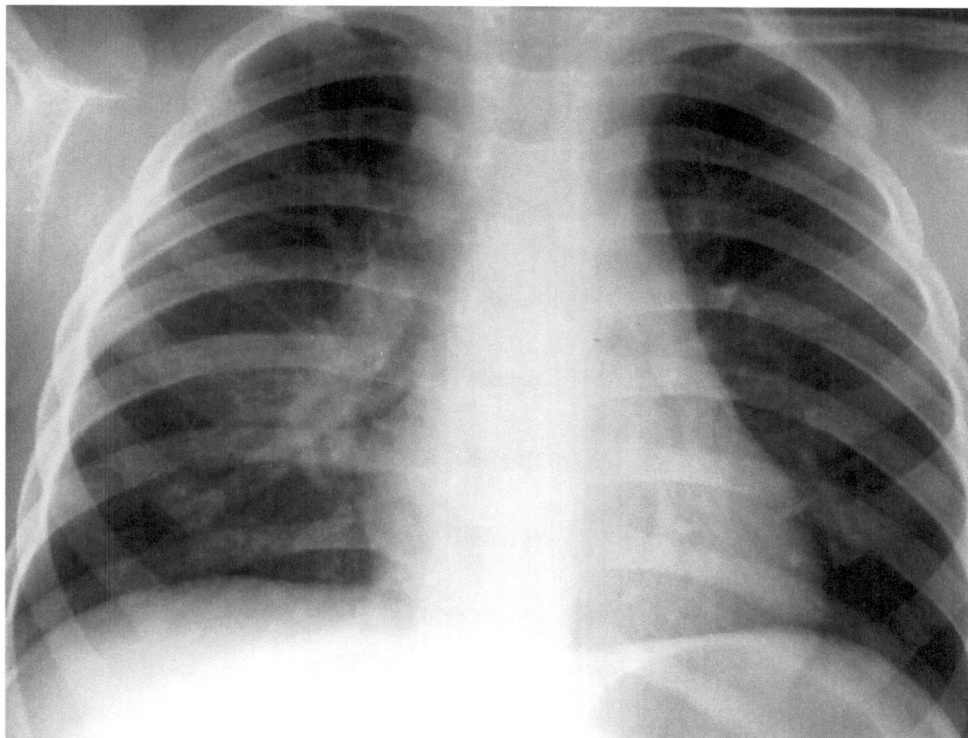

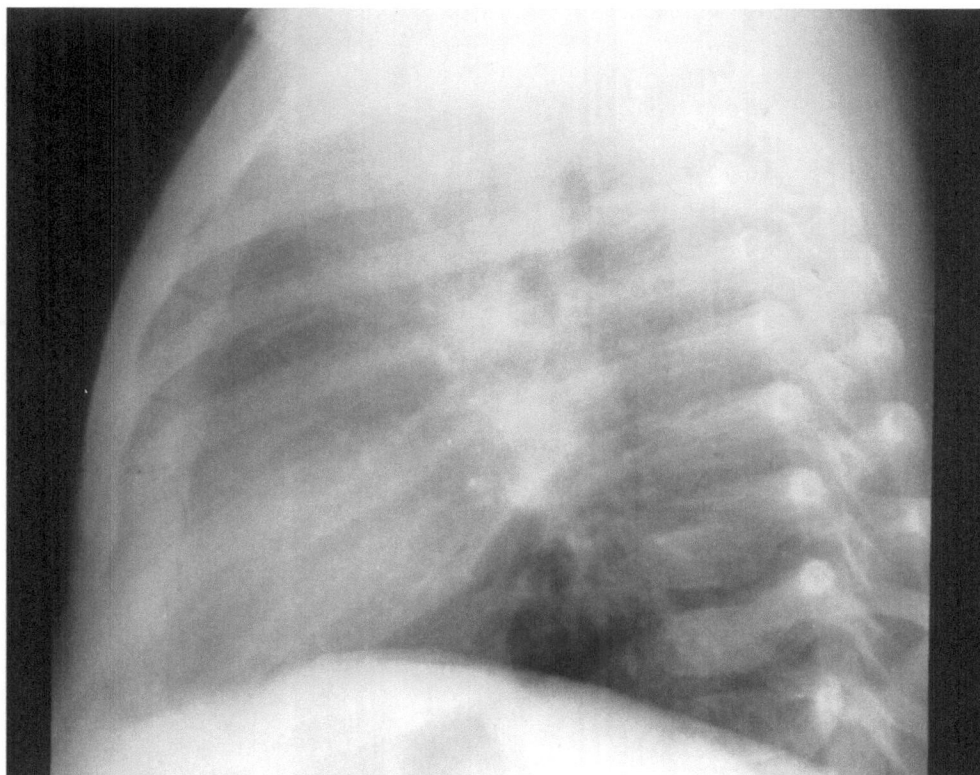

A frontal radiograph of a 4 years-old child, demonstrates right hilar and paratracheal lymphadenopathy. The lateral radiograph also demonstrates hilar adenopathy.

Source: Francis J. Curry National Tuberculosis Center.

B) COMPUTER TOMOGRAPHY (CT) SCAN IMAGE

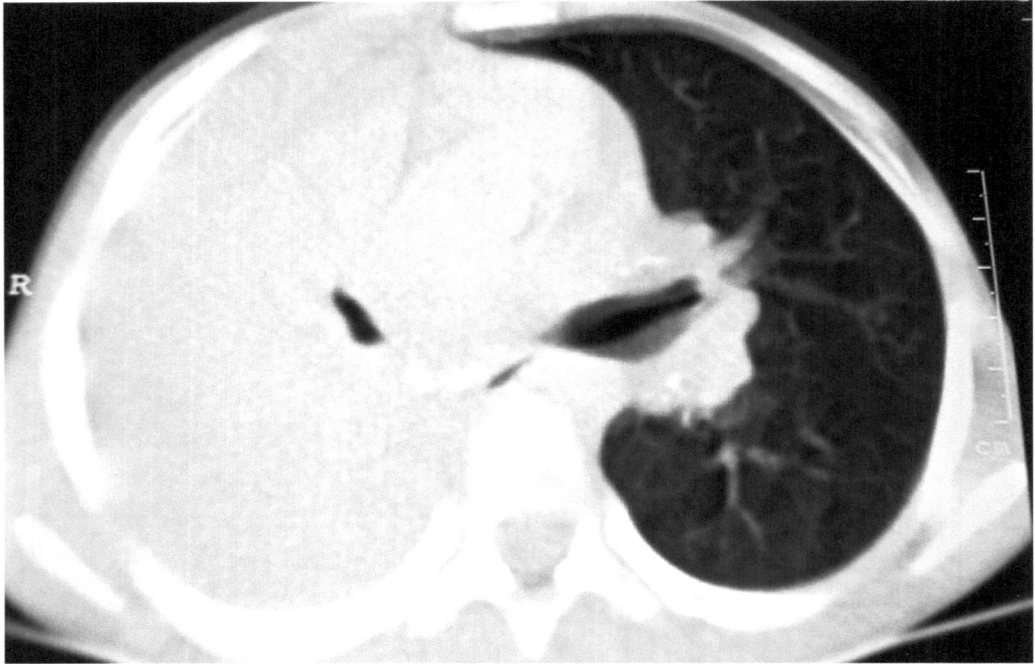

A CT scan from the same girl described earlier (see top), showing the extensive pneumonia in the right lung. Her prognosis was total atelectasis and then broncoscopy showed almost complete blockage of the right bronchi (arrow) due to extrinsical compression of the antero-medial wall by fistulae of ganglion; fistulae areas also found in the basal pyramid.

Source: Author.

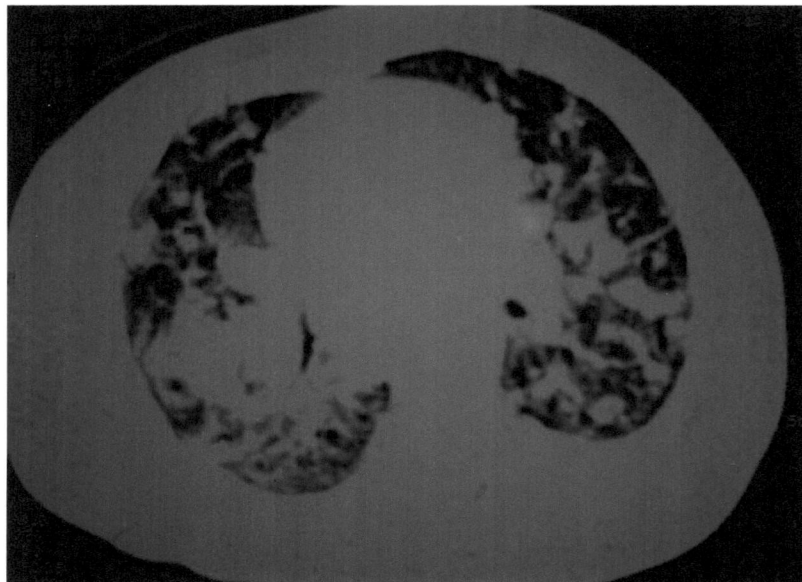

CT scan image in a 10-months boy showing airspace nodules disseminated in both lungs compatible with bronchogenic dissemination associated to areas of parenchymal consolidation in the lower lobes.

Source: Author.

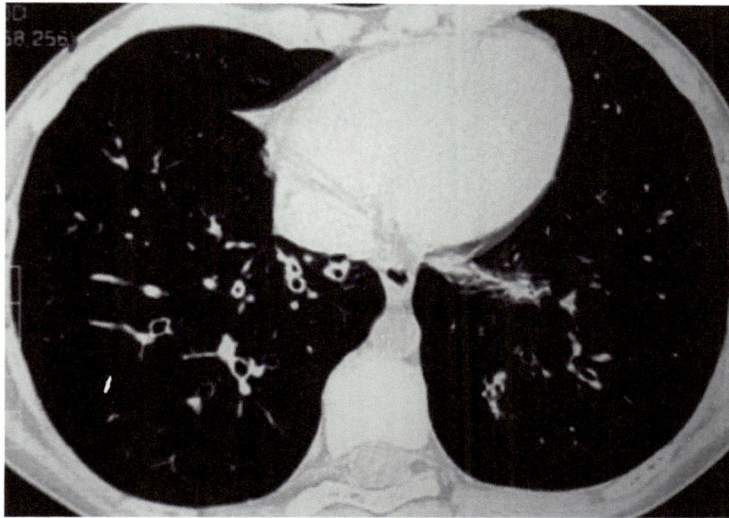

CT scan image in a 12-years old girl after treatment of tuberculosis and showing areas of bronchiectasis and segmental atelectasis.

Source: Author.

C) T-SPOT®.TB IMAGE

Patient ID	5267	5268	5270	5297	5298	5274	5309	5356	5357	5359	5370	5372	5374	5375	5376	Average
Control	0	0	0	2	0	0	0	0	0	1	0	0	0	0	0	0.2
ESAT-6	0	110	0	0	0	0	11	0	8	4	1	10	0	34	0	11.9
CFP-10	61	95	0	1	0	2	48	0	1	140	0	61	0	55	2	31.1
PHA	20	20	59	95	95	120	26	20	20	20	61	20	20	20	20	42.4
Ag85A	29	8	1	0	3	3	1	0	0	12	2	3	0	64	0	8.4
Ag85B	48	6	3	0	1	0	0	0	1	0	1	1	0	64	0	8.8
hsp65	6	1	0	0	0	2	0	1	7	0	0	2	0	4	0	1.5
Vector	0	1	0	0	0	0	0	1	0	0	1	1	0	4	1	0.5

Typical ELISpot results from individuals with suspicious tuberculosis infection. The T-SPOT®.TB commercial kit use to come with two specific *Mycobacterium tuberculosis* antigens (peptides pool), named ESAT-6 and CFP-10, plus a positive control PHA. The method was flexible enough to add other related antigens, such as Ag85A, Ag85B and hsp65, along with a negative control Vector. Number of spots of a given well is depicted in each square, and considered positive when ≥ 6.

Source: Author.

Glossary of Terms

Active tuberculosis: Currently active tuberculosis disease, whether or not it is infectious. The symptoms of disease include weakness, weight loss, fever, no appetite, chills and sweating at night. Other symptoms of tuberculosis disease depend on where in the body the bacteria are growing. If tuberculosis is in the lungs (pulmonary tuberculosis), the symptoms may include a cough, pain in the chest, and coughing up blood.

Antibiotic: A drug used to treat infections caused by bacteria and other microorganisms. Originally, an antibiotic was a substance produced by one microorganism that selectively inhibits the growth of another. Synthetic antibiotics, usually chemically related to natural antibiotics, have since been produced that accomplish comparable tasks.

Bacteria: Single-celled microorganisms which can exist either as independent (free-living) organisms or as parasites (dependent upon another organism for life).

BCG - A vaccine for tuberculosis named after the French scientists Albert Calmette and Camille Guérin. This vaccine is currently used to help prevent tuberculosis.

Breathing: The process of respiration, during which air is inhaled into the lungs through the mouth or nose due to muscle contraction, and then exhaled due to muscle relaxation.

Calcification: The process of building bone by suffusing tissues with calcium salts. Also, the image techniques may show scarring (fibrosis) or hardening (calcification) in the lungs, suggesting that the tuberculosis is contained and inactive.

Chemoprophylaxis - The administration of anti-tuberculosis drug(s) to prevent the acquisition or progression of tuberculosis infection. The former may be referred to as *primary chemoprophylaxis* or *preventive therapy*, the latter as *secondary chemoprophylaxis*.

Chest X-ray - A picture of the inside of your chest. A chest X-ray is made by exposing a film to X-rays that pass through your chest. A physician can look at this film to see whether tuberculosis bacteria have damaged your lungs.

Chest: The area of the body located between the neck and the abdomen. The chest contains the lungs, the heart and part of the aorta. The walls of the chest are supported by the dorsal vertebrae, the ribs, and the sternum.

Contact - A person who has spent time with a person with infectious tuberculosis.

Cough: A rapid expulsion of air from the lungs typically in order to clear the lung airways of fluids, mucus, or material. Also called tussis.

Culture - Tubercle bacteria in your phlegm or other body fluids are grown and identified. A culture is the propagation of microorganisms in a growth media. Any body tissue or fluid can be evaluated in the laboratory by culture techniques in order to detect and identify infectious processes. Culture techniques also be used to determine sensitivity to antibiotics.

Diagnosis: 1 The nature of a disease; the identification of an illness. **2** A conclusion or decision reached by diagnosis. The diagnosis is tuberculosis. **3** The identification of any problem.

Directly observed therapy (DOT) - A way of helping patients take their medicine for tuberculosis. If you receive DOT, you will meet with a health care worker every day or several times a week. You will meet at a place you both agree on. This can be the tuberculosis clinic, your home or work, or any other convenient

Paulo Renato Zuquim Antas, Dilvani Oliveira Santos, Roberta Olmo Pinheiro and Theolis Barbosa (Eds)

location. You will take your medicine at this place. Sometimes someone in your family or a close friend will be able to help you in a similar way to the health care worker.

Directly observed therapy, short-course (DOTS) - World Health Organization has developed a control strategy known as Directly Observed Therapy, Short-course, which requires microscopy based diagnosis, standardized treatment under direct supervision, a secure supply of quality drugs and equipment, careful monitoring and supervision, and political commitment to support these activities.

Disease: Illness or sickness often characterized by typical patient problems (symptoms) and physical findings (signs).

Extrapulmonary tuberculosis - Tuberculosis disease in any part of the body other than the lungs (such as the kidney or lymph nodes).

Fever: Although a fever technically is any body temperature above the normal of 98.6 degrees. (37 degrees C.), in practice a person is usually not considered to have a significant fever until the temperature is above 100.4 degrees (38 degrees C.).

Health: As officially defined by the World Health Organization, a state of complete physical, mental, and social well-being, not merely the absence of disease or infirmity.

HIV infection - Infection with human immunodeficiency virus, the virus that causes AIDS (acquired immunodeficiency syndrome). A person with both tuberculosis infection and HIV infection (tuberculosis and HIV co-infection) is at very high for tuberculosis disease.

Immune response: Any reaction by the immune system, which is a complex system that is responsible for distinguishing us from everything foreign to us, and for protecting us against infections and foreign substances. The immune system works to seek and kill invaders.

Infection: The growth of a parasitic organism within the body. (A parasitic organism is one that lives on or in another organism and draws its nourishment). A person with an infection has another organism (a "germ") growing within him or her, drawing its nourishment from the person.

Infectious person - A person who can spread tuberculosis to others because he or she is coughing tubercle bacteria into the air.

Infectious tuberculosis - Active tuberculosis disease which presents a risk of transmission of infection to others. For most practical purposes, this means sputum-smear-positive pulmonary tuberculosis in which acid fast bacilli (AFB) are present on direct microscopy of sputum. Disease of other parts of the respiratory tract or oral cavity, though rare, must also be considered infectious. Factors which increase infectiousness include the presence of cavities in the lungs, laryngeal tuberculosis and cough.

Isoniazid - A drug used to prevent tuberculosis disease in people who have tuberculosis infection. Isoniazid is also one of the five drugs used to treat the disease.

Laboratory: A place for doing tests and research procedures and preparing chemicals, etc. Although "laboratory" looks very like the Latin "laboratorium" (a place to labor, a work place), the word "laboratory" came from the Latin "elaborare" (to work out, as a problem, and with great pains), as evidenced by the Old English spelling "elaboratory" designating "a place where learned effort was applied to the solution of scientific problems".

Latent tuberculosis (sometimes known as 'dormant' tuberculosis): A state in which viable mycobacteria are present in the body without currently causing active disease but with the potential to reactivate and cause disease. The latent focus may be the result of tuberculosis infection which has not progressed to cause disease, or old tuberculosis disease that is not currently active, such as calcified nodes on chest X-ray. An adequate course of chemoprophylaxis (or anti-tuberculosis treatment) is believed to effectively prevent a latent focus from reactivating in most patients for at least 20 years.

Lobe: Part of an organ that appears to be separate in some way from the rest. A lobe may be demarcated from the rest of the organ by a fissure (crack), sulcus (groove), connective tissue or simply by its shape.

Lungs: The lungs are a pair of breathing organs located with the chest which remove carbon dioxide from and bring oxygen to the blood. There is a right and left lung.

Meningitis: An infection or inflammation of the membranes that cover the brain and spinal cord. It is usually caused by bacteria or a virus.

Microscope: An optical instrument that augments the power of the eye to see small objects. The name microscope was coined by Johannes Faber (1574-1629) who in 1628 borrowed from the Greek to combined micro-, small with skopein, to view. Although the first microscopes were simple microscopes, most (if not all) optical microscopes today are compound microscopes.

Multidrug-resistant tuberculosis (MDR TB) - Tuberculosis resistant to isoniazid and rifampicin, with or without any other resistance.

Mycobacteria - The genus of bacteria which includes the organisms which cause tuberculosis, but also bacteria of lower pathogenicity which are not transmitted person-to-person. It is a large family of bacteria that have unusually waxy cell walls that are resistant to digestion.

***Mycobacteria tuberculosis* complex** - A group of closely related mycobacterial species (*M. tuberculosis*, *M. bovis* and *M. africanum*) which can cause tuberculosis.

Night sweats: Severe hot flashes which occur at night and result in a drenching sweat. Night sweats can have many different causes including medications, infections, and cancers.

Old/previous tuberculosis: Tuberculosis disease which has either healed naturally or been fully treated and shows no evidence of current activity. It may or may not be latent.

PPD: Purified protein derivative (the PPD skin test for tuberculosis).

Public health: The approach to medicine that is concerned with the health of the community as a whole. Public health is community health. It has been said that: "Health care is vital to all of us some of the time, but public health is vital to all of us all of the time".

Pulmonary tuberculosis - Tuberculosis disease that occurs in the lungs, usually producing a cough that lasts longer than 2 weeks. Most tuberculosis disease is pulmonary.

Reactivated tuberculosis: Old tuberculosis infection (whether previously known or not) which has become active.

Re-infection: Active tuberculosis due to acquisition of new infection in someone who has had previous tuberculosis infection.

Resistance: Opposition to something, or the ability to withstand it. For example, some forms of tubercle bacilli are resistant to treatment with antibiotics.

Resistant bacteria - Bacteria that can no longer be killed by a certain drug.

Rifampicin - A drug used to prevent tuberculosis disease in people who have tuberculosis infection. Rifampicin is also one of the five drugs used to treat tuberculosis disease.

Sputum - The mucus and other matter brought up from the lungs, bronchi, and trachea that one may cough up and spit out or swallow. The word "sputum" is borrowed directly from the Latin "to spit." Called also expectoration. Sputum is examined for tuberculosis bacteria using a smear; part of the sputum can also be used to do a culture.

Sputum Smear - A test to see whether there are tubercle bacteria in your phlegm. To do this test, lab workers smear the phlegm on a glass slide, stain the slide with a special stain, and look for bacteria on the slide. This test usually takes one day.

Sputum smear-positive tuberculosis (sometimes called 'open' tuberculosis): Pulmonary tuberculosis in which mycobacteria ('acid-fast bacilli', AFB) have been seen in a stained smear of sputum examined under a microscope. Confirmation of the diagnosis requires culture to differentiate the organisms from atypical mycobacteria.

Tuberculin - A reagent which is derived from inactivated tubercle bacilli is injected under the skin on the lower part of your arm in doing a tuberculosis skin test. If you have tuberculosis infection, you will probably have a positive reaction to the tuberculin.

Tuberculin skin tests - A skin test is carried out to determine if you may have been infected with tuberculosis. These are generally referred to as 'positive' or 'negative'. It is also called as Pirquet, PPD or Mantoux test, named for the French physician Charles Mantoux (1877-1947).

Tuberculosis (TB): Disease due to infection with *Mycobacterium tuberculosis* complex.

Tuberculosis infection: A condition in which *M. tuberculosis* organisms are present in the body without necessarily causing active tuberculosis *disease*.

Weight loss: A decrease in body weight resulting from either voluntary (diet, exercise) or involuntary (illness) circumstances. Most instances of weight loss arise due to the loss of body fat, but in cases of extreme or severe weight loss, protein and other substances in the body can also be depleted.

Index

A

Acid-fast bacilli (AFB) 2, 79, 81-84, 92, 103, 124-127
Albert Calmette 14
Albert Schatz 14
Alexandre Dumas 13
Alveolar macrophages 23, 24, 56

B

Bacillus Calmette Guérin (BCG) vaccine 11-14, 26, 29, 37, 54, 55, 60-63, *74*, 87-91, *130*, 136, 138-142
Breastfeeding *170*, *173*
Bronchial 20, *78*, *81*, 102, 104, 112-115, *130*, 135
Bronchiectasis 76, 83, 103, 105, 112-115
Bronchoscopy (in video available)

C

Caelius Aurelianus 8
Camille Guérin 15
Carlo Forlanini 12
Chest radiography 2, *8*, 19, *21*, 25, 28, 41, 55, *74*, 76, 77, *89*, 100-115, 118, 125, 140
Co-infection (see HIV infection)
Computed tomography (CT) 76, 77, 100, 105, *109*, 112-118
Cough 19, 25, 31, *74*, 75, *81*, 160
Cytokines 24, 54-57, 60, 61, 138, 139

D

Diagnosis 1, 2, 6, 19, 28, 34, 39-41, 47, 53-55, 63, 73-78, 83, 85, 86, 89-93, 100-106, 113-119, 123-126, 131, 136-138, 141, 142, 160-163
Drug resistance 10, 29, 35, 45, 46, 54, 84, 117, 132, 134, 163

E

Edward Livingston Trudeau 12
Empyema 108, *109*
Epidemiology 18, 34, 35, 43, 45, 73
Extensive drug resistant tuberculosis (see Drug resistance)

F

Fibrosis 83, 105, 111, 112

G

George Bodington 9
Gerhard Domagk 14
Ghon focus 2, 19-21, 102
Giacomo Puccini 13
Gibbous deformity (see Pott's disease)
Giuseppe Verdi 13
Granuloma 3, *25*, 56, 61, 77, 102

Paulo Renato Zuquim Antas, Dilvani Oliveira Santos, Roberta Olmo Pinheiro and Theolis Barbosa (Eds)

H

Hermann Brehmer 12
Hippocrates 7, 8
HIV infection 3, 22, 29, 30, 34, 35, 39, 40, 44, 45, 61, 62, 73, 74, 76, 82, 88-91, 100, 110, 115, 116, 124,
        125, 131, 135-137, 140, 142, 159, 162, *163*
Holger Mollgaard 13

I

Imaging techniques 27, 124, 161
Immunosuppression 62, 63, 110, 115, 159
Interleukins 24, 57

J

Jean Antoine Villemin 9
Johann Lukas Schönlein 8
John Crofton 15
John Keats 13
Jörgen Lehmann 14

K

Kinyoun (see acid-fast bacilli)

L

Lipoarabinomanann (LAM) 57, 58, 135-138, 153
Lymphadenitis (Tuberculous lymphadenitis) 91, 102, 126, 131
Lymphocytes 23, 54, 58-62, 70, 76, 93, 99, 101, 115

M

Mantoux test (see Tuberculin Skin Test)
Meningitis (Tuberculous meningitis) 3, 28-31, *38*, 39, 43, 44, 46, 76, 77, 92, 125, 131, 142,
Multiple drug resistant tuberculosis (see Drug resistance)

N

Neutrophils 23, 56, *59*, 76, 93
Nitric oxide 57
Nocard 10

P

Pasteur 9, 11
Paul Ehrlich 4
Pirquet test (see Tuberculin Skin Test)
Pleural effusions 20, 77, 101, 103, 106, 108, *109*, 111
Pneumonia 39, 46, 73, 75-78, 104
Polymerase Chain Reaction (PCR) 93, 129-133, 160, 161
Pott's disease 7, 75
Purified Protein Derivative (PPD) 6, 11, 20, 55, 87, 88, 89

R

René Théophile Hyacinthe Laennec 8